COUNTY DISTRICT LIBRARY
230 E. MAIN STREET
LOGAN, OHIO 43138

Lynette S. Chandler
Shelly J. Lane
Editors

Children with Prenatal Drug Exposure

D0144145

Pre-publication
REVIEWS,
COMMENTARIES,
EVALUATIONS . . .

"**T**his book gives a very comprehensive view of the available literature regarding children prenatally exposed to drugs. In doing so, it sheds light on the overlapping issues affecting infants and their families which, if not dealt with, will negatively affect any intervention.

An up-to-date test which will be most helpful to all practitioners who work with children prenatally exposed to drugs."

Helmi Owens, EdD
Professor of Special Education
Pacific Lutheran University
Tacoma, Washington

More pre-publication
REVIEWS, COMMENTARIES, EVALUATIONS . . .

"**T**he subject of prenatal exposure to drugs is a very pertinent one in the current era and one that begs for a foundation of research and scholarly endeavors. To start the book out with a writing directed to the ethics surrounding this subject, raised my consciousness toward the complexities of dealing with mothers and children in these circumstances. The results of ongoing research are vital to the further development of a body of knowledge in this area and should serve as an excellent resource for practitioners in the field interested in this topic. A great follow-up to this publication would be one which further focuses on the application of the research materials to practice. I hope this is a catalyst for future publications dealing with the wide-range impact of prenatal drug exposure."

Denise A. Rotert, MA, OTR/L
Associate Professor, Department of Occupational Therapy University of South Dakota

"**T**his book is a compilation of research articles by different authors who have investigated the effects that various drugs have on fetuses (emphasis is on crack/cocaine) coupled with follow-up studies of various performance measures of drug exposed infants and children compared to normed populations.

Therapists, doctors, nurses and those in our educational systems will find this book of value for updating their knowledge on current research findings concerning fetuses exposed to drugs in utero as well as clearly stating the pros and cons of the effects that this exposure has on the behaviors of these infants and children. Fortunately, many of the authors of this book point out the problems involved when doing research on the polydrug effects on the developing fetus as well as working with the drug addicted mother or parent who is in a recovery program, while trying to care for her drug exposed infant. This book is excellent for pointing out all of the multifactorial parameters that must be considered when working with these infants/children and their caretakers, and/or doing research on the effects of polydrug use on fetuses and investigating the unknown future potentials of these exposed individuals.

More pre-publication
REVIEWS, COMMENTARIES, EVALUATIONS . . .

Another value of this publication concerns the use of various normed tests and measurements available to researchers who study infants, young children and middle-aged children who have, or have not, been exposed to polydrugs in utero. The reader will gain excellent insight into many of these tests, how they are used and the results that can be obtained within the limits of these various tests.

Many authors stress the need for additional research, especially in critical areas where knowledge is lacking, as to the long term effects of perinatal drug exposure, postnatal development and especially long term or longitudinal follow-up studies. If anyone is in doubt as to "what to research next" this complication opens the mind to hundreds of research projects waiting to be researched, especially by those who work with this growing population of polydrug exposed infants, children, teenagers and parents."

Josephine C. Moore, PhD OTR, DSc (Hon)[2], FAOTA
Professor Emeritus, Department of Anatomy, University of South Dakota Medical School, Vermillion

The Haworth Press, Inc.

Children with Prenatal Drug Exposure

ALL HAWORTH BOOKS AND JOURNALS
ARE PRINTED ON CERTIFIED
ACID-FREE PAPER

Children with Prenatal Drug Exposure

Lynette S. Chandler
Shelly J. Lane
Editors

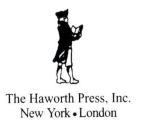

The Haworth Press, Inc.
New York • London

Children with Prenatal Drug Exposure has also been published as *Physical & Occupational Therapy in Pediatrics*, Volume 16, Numbers 1/2 1996.

© 1996 by The Haworth Press, Inc. All rights reserved. No part of this work may be reproduced or utilized in any form or by any means, electronic or mechanical, including photocopying, microfilm and recording, or by any information storage and retrieval system, without permission in writing from the publisher. Printed in the United States of America.

The Haworth Press, Inc., 10 Alice Street, Binghamton, NY 13904-1580 USA

Paperback edition published in 1997.

Cover design by Maria Vail.

Library of Congress Cataloging-in-Publication Data

Children with prenatal drug exposure / Lynette S. Chandler, Shelly J. Lane, editors.
    p. cm.
Includes bibliographical references and index.
ISBN 0-7890-0221-3 (alk. paper)
    1. Children of prenatal substance abuse. I. Chandler, Lynette S. II. Lane, Shelly J.
RJ520.P74C47 1996
618.92'86–dc20   96-19136
                                                                   CIP

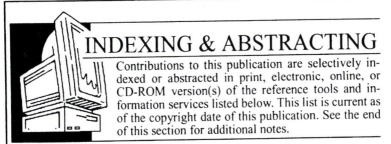

INDEXING & ABSTRACTING

Contributions to this publication are selectively indexed or abstracted in print, electronic, online, or CD-ROM version(s) of the reference tools and information services listed below. This list is current as of the copyright date of this publication. See the end of this section for additional notes.

- *Academic Abstracts/CD-ROM,* EBSCO Publishing, P.O. Box 2250, Peabody, MA 01960-7250

- *Biosciences Information Service of Biological Abstracts (BIOSIS),* Biosciences Information Service, 2100 Arch Street, Philadelphia, PA 19103-1399

- *Child Development Abstracts & Bibliography,* University of Kansas, 2 Bailey Hall, Lawrence, KS 66045

- *CINAHL (Cumulative Index to Nursing & Allied Health Literature), in print, also on CD-ROM from CD PLUS, EBSCO, and SilverPlatter, and online from CDP Online (formerly BRS), Data-Star, and PaperChase. (Support materials include Subject Heading List, Database Search Guide, and instructional video),* CINAHL Information Systems, P.O. Box 871/1509 Wilson Terrace, Glendale, CA 91209-0871

- *CNPIEC Reference Guide: Chinese National Directory of Foreign Periodicals,* P.O. Box 88, Beijing, People's Republic of China

- *Developmental Medicine & Child Neurology,* Mac Keith Press, 526-529 High Holborn House, 52-54 High Holborn, London WC1V 6RL, England

- *Educational Administration Abstracts (EAA),* Sage Publications, Inc., 2455 Teller Road, Newbury Park, CA 91320

- *Exceptional Child Education Resources (ECER), (online through DIALOG and hard copy),* The Council for Exceptional Children, 1920 Association Drive, Reston, VA 22091

(continued)

- *Excerpta Medica/Secondary Publishing Division,* Elsevier Science Inc., Secondary Publishing Division, 655 Avenue of the Americas, New York, NY 10010

- *Family Studies Database (online and CD/ROM),* Peters Technology Transfer, 306 East Baltimore Pike, 2nd Floor, Media, PA 19063

- *Health Source: Indexing & Abstracting of 160 selected health related journals, updated monthly:* EBSCO Publishing, 83 Pine Street, Peabody, MA 01960

- *Health Source Plus: expanded version of "Health Source" to be released shortly:* EBSCO Publishing, 83 Pine Street, Peabody, MA 01960

- *INTERNET ACCESS (& additional networks) Bulletin Board for Libraries ("BUBL"), coverage of information resources on INTERNET, JANET, and other networks.*
  - JANET X.29: UK.AC.BATH.BUBL or 00006012101300
  - TELNET: BUBL.BATH.AC.UK or 138.38.32.45 login 'bubl'
  - Gopher: BUBL.BATH.AC.UK (138.32.32.45). Port 7070
  - World Wide Web: http://www.bubl.bath.ac.uk./BUBL/home.html
  - NISSWAIS: telnetniss.ac.uk (for the NISS gateway)
  The Andersonian Library, Curran Building, 101 St. James Road, Glasgow G4 ONS, Scotland

- *Occupational Therapy Database (OTDBASE),* 3485 Point Grey Road, Vancouver, BC V6R 1A6, Canada

- *Occupational Therapy Index,* British Library Medical Information Service, Boston Spa, Wetherby, West Yorkshire, LS23 7BQ, United Kingdom

- *OT BibSys,* American Occupational Therapy Foundation, P.O. Box 31220, Rockville, MD 20824-1220

- *Sage Family Studies Abstracts (SFSA),* Sage Publications, Inc., 2455 Teller Road, Newbury Park, CA 91320

- *Sage Urban Studies Abstracts (SUSA),* Sage Publications, Inc., 2455 Teller Road, Newbury Park, CA 91320

(continued)

- *Social Work Abstracts,* National Association of Social Workers, 750 First Street NW, 8th Floor, Washington, DC 20002

- *Sport Database/Discus,* Sport Information Resource Center, 1600 James Naismith Drive, Suite 107, Gloucester, Ontario K1B 5N4, Canada

- *Violence and Abuse Abstracts: A Review of Current Literature on Interpersonal Violence (VAA),* Sage Publications, Inc., 2455 Teller Road, Newbury Park, CA 91320

SPECIAL BIBLIOGRAPHIC NOTES

related to special journal issues (separates)
and indexing/abstracting

☐ indexing/abstracting services in this list will also cover material in any "separate" that is co-published simultaneously with Haworth's special thematic journal issue or DocuSerial. Indexing/abstracting usually covers material at the article/chapter level.

☐ monographic co-editions are intended for either non-subscribers or libraries which intend to purchase a second copy for their circulating collections.

☐ monographic co-editions are reported to all jobbers/wholesalers/approval plans. The source journal is listed as the "series" to assist the prevention of duplicate purchasing in the same manner utilized for books-in-series.

☐ to facilitate user/access services all indexing/abstracting services are encouraged to utilize the co-indexing entry note indicated at the bottom of the first page of each article/chapter/contribution.

☐ this is intended to assist a library user of any reference tool (whether print, electronic, online, or CD-ROM) to locate the monographic version if the library has purchased this version but not a subscription to the source journal.

☐ individual articles/chapters in any Haworth publication are also available through the Haworth Document Delivery Services (HDDS).

Children with Prenatal Drug Exposure

CONTENTS

ABOUT THE EDITORS

Lynette S. Chandler, PhD, PT, is Professor of Physical Therapy at the University of Puget Sound in Tacoma, Washington. For many years she served as a clinician for children in a variety of settings, including a rehabilitation center, homes, schools, and at the Clinical Research Center at the University of Washington. It was while Dr. Chandler was working on her Bachelor's degree at Simmons College and working at the Children's Hospital in Boston that she first became aware of the need for and realities of assessment of infants. Particularly interested in the effects of prenatal exposure to drugs, Dr. Chandler continues an affiliation with the University of Pittsburgh, where she has completed an analytical study of more than 500 three-year-olds.

Shelly J. Lane, PhD, OTR/L, FAOTA, is Assistant Professor of Occupational Therapy at the State University of New York at Buffalo. Formerly Assistant Professor at the University of Alabama at Birmingham and Director of Occupational Therapy at the Sparks Center, Dr. Lane's specialization in pediatrics began while working with preschool and elementary school children in both public and private schools in Kentucky. Her research interests while pursuing her PhD in Anatomy and Neuroscience and later while holding a postdoctural fellowship at the Neuropsychiatric Institute at UCLA included the effects of barbiturate dependence and withdrawal on neurotransmitters and second messenger systems within the cerebellum and the acoustic startle response in typical children and children with autism and attention deficit disorder. Recently, she has conducted research studies on the sensory and motor development in four-year-old children born prematurely, the interrater reliability of a newborn assessment tool, and long-term development of infants and children exposed to cocaine *in utero*. Dr. Lane is currently Project Director for "Let's Play!", a model demonstration project which is parent-driven and capitalizes on assistive technology to promote play for very young children with disabilities and their families.

Introduction

Lynette S. Chandler
Shelly J. Lane

Most of the authors in this special volume are intimately involved as clinicians in the care of the children prenatally exposed to drugs and their families. Their concerns have led them beyond their roles as clinicians into their roles as researchers. The data generated by their ongoing research will help clinicians to promote the health of children and their families. Their research should entice the clinicians among us to document systematically our assessments and treatments for later analysis of the effect of treatment.

We have begun this special volume with the ethics of care. Mattingly has written an article that demands your thoughtful consideration. She carefully and clearly articulates the dilemma for health professionals as "how to act vigorously to protect and promote child health without treating pregnant women and mothers in ways that are ultimately unfair or counterproductive."

Lane summarizes the actions of cocaine and the implications of its use. The complexity of research in the arena of prenatal cocaine exposure becomes clear as each variable is discussed including, for example, the impact of pattern of use, withdrawal, and paternal contribution.

A complete and thorough discussion of the evaluation of neuromotor outcomes of infants exposed to cocaine by Swanson ends with a concise review of the neuromotor outcomes of prenatal exposure to cocaine as supported by rigorous scientific procedure. Intervention, according to Swanson, must be individualized and realistic, taking into consideration the potential for a positive outcome.

[Haworth co-indexing entry note]: "Introduction." Chandler, Lynette S., and Shelly J. Lane. Co-published simultaneously in *Physical & Occupational Therapy in Pediatrics* (The Haworth Press, Inc.) Vol. 16, No. 1/2, 1996, pp. 1-3; and: *Children with Prenatal Drug Exposure* (ed: Lynette S. Chandler, and Shelly J. Lane) The Haworth Press, Inc., 1996, pp. 1-3. Single or multiple copies of this article are available from The Haworth Document Delivery Service [1-800-342-9678, 9:00 a.m. - 5:00 p.m. (EST). E-mail address: getinfo@haworth.com].

© 1996 by The Haworth Press, Inc. All rights reserved. *1*

Stewart, Richardson, and Olson describe the MOM's Project, which was designed to investigate comprehensive services to chemically-dependent pregnant women and their children. The emphasis of this article is on the transactional model of development used to assess children who have been prenatally exposed to alcohol or illicit drugs. The system used by the MOM's project to assess the quality of infant development and to assess caregiver-infant interaction evolved from a thoughtful review of the multifaceted problems facing clinicians and researchers. Suggestions for future directions in research should provide the clinician/researcher some direction for his or her own work.

Rose-Jacobs, Frank, and Brown continue the discussion of issues of measurement. Though there is certainly overlap in some of the assessments discussed by the authors of the two preceding articles, you will no doubt find that each article is unique unto itself, expressing the diverse experience of each researcher. These authors call for multidimensional measurement systems which can be used in longitudinal research.

Arendt, Minnes, and Singer integrate the results of their research with that of previously published research. The emphasis for this article is on the neurologic effects and sensory motor delays of cocaine exposure. They give suggestions for intervention.

Bayer, Bleichfeld, Lane, Volker, Alif, and Floss examined the relationship between motor performance as measured by the Movement Assessment of Infants (MAI) with novelty preference scores of the Fagan Test of Infant Intelligence (FTII) on children previously exposed to cocaine in utero. Thirty-six full term infants were assessed at eight months (MAI) and 69 weeks (FTII). The interesting results are discussed in the context of a homeostatic model of functioning.

Adolescent pregnancy and the complications of prenatal substance use is the focus of another article. Cornelius postulates, as the result of the analysis of data on the offspring of 310 teenagers, that young maternal age may increase the risk of negative effects of tobacco, alcohol, and marijuana for the neonate. Given the increasing rate of teenage pregnancies, this research makes an invaluable contribution to the understanding of the complex issues surrounding prenatal substance exposure.

Grattan and Hans have followed children prenatally exposed to opiates (heroin and methadone) from birth to ten years of age. The article in this book reports on the motor assessment of children who were nine to eleven years of age at the time of their assessment. Children with documented histories of prenatal exposure to opioids are compared with children with no history of prenatal substance exposure. This longitudinal study adds a critical component to our understanding of prenatal exposure to drugs, in this case, opioids.

Giusti's research focuses on 24 children in foster care. The children included drug-exposed and non-exposed children. Giusti's study gives credence to the thought that treatment solutions are not easy to find. Solutions that we use, however, must be subjected to careful documentation and analysis.

The final article by Riegger-Krugh, Blair, and Sparling is unique within this volume. The researchers use video-computer technology and real-time ultrasound to study fetal knee angular velocity. Two fetuses are studied, one whose mother was cocaine addicted during the pregnancy and one whose mother did not use cocaine. The methodological process used in this study is challenging and innovative. It should be of interest to all of us.

We trust that the readers will enjoy reading and analyzing the articles in this volume as much as we have as guest editors. The authors have been generous in sharing their research with us, sometimes research which is still in progress. We thank them for their suggestions for assessment, treatment and further research.

The Mother-Fetal Dyad
and the Ethics of Care

Susan S. Mattingly

SUMMARY. Increasing knowledge of the effects on infants of mothers' behaviors during pregnancy raises important ethical issues for health professionals regarding their moral obligations and appropriate responses. This paper reviews the flaws in applying the two-patient (mother and fetus) model of medical care to the ethical dilemmas involved in efforts to prevent or reduce morbidity in offspring. A more appropriate ethical response combines clinical efforts to alter maternal behavior with attention to maternal support systems and public policy advocacy to create an environment more conducive to health and parental responsibility. *[Article copies available from The Haworth Document Delivery Service: 1-800-342-9678. E-mail address: getinfo@haworth.com]*

A rapidly growing body of knowledge is increasing our understanding and awareness of links between neonatal pathologies and the mother's behavior during, and even prior to, pregnancy. With increasing precision and certainty, maternal factors such as malnutrition, drug use, smoking, and exposure to workplace hazards are being identified as measurable contributors to infant morbidity.

Health professionals who struggle daily with the tragic consequences of unhealthy maternal choices see the preventable illness of infants and children not only as a health problem but as an ethical problem of major

---

Susan S. Mattingly, PhD, is Professor of Philosophy, Lincoln University, Jefferson City, MO 65102.

[Haworth co-indexing entry note]: "The Mother-Fetal Dyad and the Ethics of Care." Mattingly, Susan S. Co-published simultaneously in *Physical & Occupational Therapy in Pediatrics* (The Haworth Press, Inc.) Vol. 16, No. 1/2, 1996, pp. 5-13; and: *Children with Prenatal Drug Exposure* (ed: Lynette S. Chandler, and Shelly J. Lane) The Haworth Press, Inc., 1996, pp. 5-13. Single or multiple copies of this article are available from The Haworth Document Delivery Service [1-800-342-9678, 9:00 a.m. - 5:00 p.m. (EST). E-mail address: getinfo@haworth.com].

© 1996 by The Haworth Press, Inc. All rights reserved.

proportions. Analyzing that problem, identifying all of the relevant moral obligations, and, especially, determining what response is consistent with professional ethics are tasks that are surprisingly complex.

Although the mother's behavior is the proximate cause of many perinatal harms, that behavior occurs in a broader social context, and it is important to consider what other contributing factors may be implicated. Are there other moral agents who share responsibility for fetal health? If so, what are the various obligations and how are they distributed? Furthermore, efforts to change maternal behaviors must be sensitive to the standards and values of the health professions. What limits are implied by the mother's status as a patient or client? What are the likely long-term consequences for this child, and for children in general? The ethical dilemma for health professionals is how to act vigorously to protect and promote child health without treating pregnant women and mothers in ways that are ultimately unfair or counterproductive.

THE TWO-PATIENT MODEL AND THE ETHICS OF CONFLICTING RIGHTS

Unfortunately, the problem of perinatal health risks is usually cast as a conflict between maternal and fetal rights, an oversimplification that slants the issue and obscures many interesting and important questions. This way of defining the ethical problem derives an aura of authority from the new two-patient medical model of the mother-fetus dyad. Traditionally, obstetricians conceptualized the mother-fetal dyad as one patient, the pregnant woman.[1,2] The fetus was not sharply distinguished from the mother's condition of pregnancy. In the interests of the pregnant woman's health, physicians provided patient education and advocated behaviors to reduce risks. In so doing, physicians acted under the ethical principle of *beneficence:* the fundamental professional duty to do good and avoid harm, to promote the patient's health, and to protect her from illness and injury.[3] The important point to note is that in the one-patient model, the pregnant woman's health *included* the health of her pregnancy. Thus, behaviors that posed fetal risks were thought of and presented as being harmful to her (them), while more healthful habits were recommended and urged for her (their) good. Singular and plural, self and other, tend to blur in the unity of the one-patient mother-fetal dyad.

The two-patient model represents a conceptual shift in obstetric medicine in response to diagnostic and treatment developments that now, for the first time, allow physicians to interact directly with the fetus. Ultrasonography, techniques for sampling fetal tissues, and *in utero* therapeutic procedures have transformed the fetus into a second patient, distinct from the mother. The mother is the site of these medical interactions, of course, but she is no longer viewed as the essential medium through which the fetus is indirectly known and affected. She remains a patient with her own distinctive medical needs, but in terms of the physician-fetus relationship, she has become transparent. For the physician, the "oneness" of the mother-fetal dyad has dissipated, and its "twoness" has crystallized into a framework for clinical practice.[1,2]

The two-patient obstetric model is being used, rather uncritically, in my opinion, to redefine the ethics of perinatal patient care. Conceptually dividing the pregnant woman into two patients is assumed to create a new set of ethical relationships between and among mother, fetus, and physician.[4-6] The argument goes something like this: First, if the fetus is medically treatable as a distinct individual patient, then the fetus must possess all of the moral rights associated with individuality, including the right not to be harmed. This is a strong moral right that admits very few justifiable exceptions. Second, if the fetus has a moral right not to be harmed, then the mother has a moral obligation to the fetus to avoid risky personal behaviors. Because the right against harm is very strong, the corresponding duty not to harm is extremely stringent as well. Third, if the fetus is an individual patient with moral rights, then the physician has a duty, under the principle of beneficence, to protect the fetal patient's health. This duty is independent of professional duties to the maternal patient and may, in fact, occasionally come into conflict with them.

This analysis depicts the problem of high-risk maternal activities as a conflict between the fetus's moral right not to be harmed and the mother's right to choose her own behavior, with the medical professional thrust into the role of referee. Because the right against harm, the obligation not to harm, and the duty to protect patients against harm are fundamental ethical rights and duties, this way of defining the problem virtually assures judgments in favor of the fetus. Only if the mother's own rights against harm were at stake would there be a difficult balancing decision to make. For example, when a pregnant women is suffering from severe depression, a physician might prescribe medications for her even though they entail some risk of fetal abnormality. Given two beneficence duties—to protect the health of the mother and to protect the health of the fetus—a physician may reasonably judge that maternal treatment represents an acceptable compromise, particularly as he or she thinks ahead to the woman's ability to care for her baby after birth. Health benefits for the mother usually contribute to the child's best interests as well, thus offsetting small increases in risks.

On the other hand, when perinatal risks are imposed by the mother's use of illicit drugs or other behavior that is potentially harmful to her own health as well as that of the fetus, there is, according to the "conflicting rights" analysis, no real dilemma for the professional. The mother's right in this instance is not the strong right against being harmed but the relatively weaker right of *autonomy*: the right to be at liberty in making one's own choices and in living one's own life.[3] This right is limited by the *harm principle*: a competent individual is morally free to do as she pleases, even if her actions are likely to harm herself, but the right of autonomy does not extend to choices and actions that are likely to cause harm to others. Consequently, looking at the situation from the professional's viewpoint, the conflict for the professional is between a *beneficence duty to the fetus* and a *duty to respect the mother's autonomy*. The latter duty, however, is apparently nullified in this case because the mother is not morally free to cause harm to her fetus.

The conclusion drawn from this line of reasoning is that physicians and other health professionals may and should intervene to rescue the fetus from health risks imposed by the mother. Compulsory Cesarean deliveries, mandated inpatient detoxification treatments, even coerced sterilizations or abortions, could be justified by this expansive interpretation of a fetal-protective professional ethical role.

CRITIQUE OF THE ADVERSARIAL RIGHTS-BASED MODEL

In spite of the superficial plausibility of the argument outlined above, the reasoning from the two-patient mother-fetal model to an enforcement role for health professionals is flawed. I will briefly mention two errors without dwelling on them greatly, because I see these flaws as symptoms of a deeper error, that being the mistake of trying to analyze and resolve what is essentially a public health crisis exclusively in terms of individual morality.

The previously mentioned first assumption states: "If the fetus is medically treatable as a distinct individual patient, then the fetus must possess all of the moral rights associated with individuality, including the right not to be harmed." This inference commits the fallacy of deriving a statement of value from a statement of value-free fact. The philosopher David Hume called this the *"is-ought" fallacy*.[7] Hume's point was that value judgments can never be verified by science alone but must be justified pragmatically by considering how well a system of values helps us toward commonly held preferences and goals. If the goal is to reduce the incidence of perinatal morbidity, then the relevant question is whether attributing individual rights to the fetus will contribute to that goal. From facts about what *is* now medically possible, nothing at all follows about what *ought* to be done.

Assumption 2 states: "If the fetus has a moral right not to be harmed, then the mother has an extremely stringent moral obligation to the fetus to avoid risky personal behaviors." If (for the sake of argument) we suppose that the fetus does possess individual rights, what maternal duties would they imply? Rights always imply obligations or duties, for it would be meaningless to have a right that no one had a duty to respect. But duties vary in types and stringencies. The duty to avoid harming the fetus is typically presented as if it were a *negative duty* of noninterference, so-called because fulfilling the duty requires only the negative action (or non-action) of leaving the other person alone.[8] If you are reading in the library, every person there has a negative duty (for instance) *not* to break your ribs. This duty is extremely strong in part because your right against injury is strong but also because others can so easily respect it. Unlike *positive duties* to provide benefits, negative duties entail no costs that would weigh against their performance, nor do they conflict with one another (one cannot give food to every hungry person, but one *can* simultaneously *not* break the ribs of *everyone*). This is why the negative duties are subject to almost no exceptions and no excuses.

But duties to avoid harming others are not always so easily fulfilled. If, while reading in the library, you suddenly collapse and the EMT crew is called, they will pound and compress your chest, clearly placing you at risk for a broken rib, yet they violate no moral duty. Health professionals are obligated to avoid harming their patients not by leaving them alone but by exercising due care in the course of fulfilling *positive duties* to help. Analogously, for nine months the pregnant woman *cannot* fulfill her obligations not to harm the fetus simply by leaving the fetus alone. Avoiding injury requires that she exercise due care in the course of providing positive benefits.

Duties of due care are weaker than those of noninterference to the extent that their exercise requires investments of attention, energy and resources and to the degree that risk-avoidance competes with other moral claims: Should a woman continue as long as possible in her job as an X-ray technician, risking injury to the fetus, or should she remain economically dependent on an abusive husband who threatens the well being of the child as well as herself? Should she enter a residential drug-dependency program, or should she fulfill obligations of daily care for her other children, fighting the drug problem less effectively on her own? In contexts of scarce resources and multiple responsibilities, avoiding risks is more complicated than just saying "no."

Despite the increased room for exceptions and excuses, I have no wish to deny that flagrant breaches of due care are serious wrongs. If the EMTs break your ribs by performing chest compressions carelessly because they were drinking on the job, they are guilty of malpractice. What complicates the picture in the case of pregnancy is that the mother's job allows absolutely no time off for indulging her bad habits harmlessly. Many people, including not a few health professionals, have smoking, drinking or other drug-use habits that they control sufficiently to perform work and home responsibilities without placing others at undue risk, thus meeting prevailing standards of "due care." The global nature of the responsibilities of pregnancy make them difficult to live up to. Duties of risk-avoidance during pregnancy are very far from the easy negative duties of "leaving alone."

It is sometimes argued that a woman's right to abortion allows her to escape the duties of pregnancy if she finds them onerous, therefore failure to obtain a timely abortion implies that she has voluntarily accepted them.[9] That neat theory ignores the many economic, geographic and other obstacles to abortion. It also fails to consider the force of social taboos and psychological mechanisms of denial and deferral. To a woman who cannot bring herself to end an unwanted pregnancy by choosing abortion, fetal distress and the prospect of miscarriage or stillbirth may be seen as blessings in disguise. (Similarly, health professionals caring for dying patients often prefer to distance themselves from being the cause of death: e.g., a nurse who could not remove a feeding tube is relieved when it falls out and does not hasten to replace it.)

NEEDS AND OBLIGATIONS OF CARE
IN AN ETHICAL ECOSYSTEM

The connection between maternal behaviors and perinatal risks is an urgent problem of medical ethics, but for theoretical and practical reasons, the rights-based analysis is not, I believe, a helpful way to understand it or think about solving it. Theoretically, the ethics of rights is ill-suited to resolve issues that arise in the intimacy of the family and that involve relationships of dependency and inequality. The concept of individual moral rights, with its roots in the eighteenth-century enlightenment period, was devised to explain and justify ethical obligations between individuals in the new constitutional democracies, individuals who are by hypothesis independent and equal, *not* bound to one another by preexisting ties of family, clan, tribe, rank or class. The ethics of rights is designed to regulate interactions between strangers as they enter into voluntary, reciprocal relationships for mutual advantage.

In practical terms, an adversarial rights-based model for ethical perinatal care is not well-suited to promote the long-term goal of improved infant and child health in the population at large. Unless parental ties are to be dissolved, a professional approach that exacerbates maternal hostility is unlikely to work to the child's advantage in the long run. Although coercion, or the threat of coercion, may rescue the occasional fetus, it will discourage many women from seeking prenatal medical care. An ethical analysis of perinatal care must be grounded in the distinctive characteristics of the maternal-fetal relationship, and it must look beyond medical goals of short-term rescue to broader aims of healthy children in nurturing families.

The salient characteristics of the mother-fetus relationship are intimacy, dependency and inequality. If new medical technologies make it no longer accurate to describe the mother-fetal dyad as one, the old biological fact of incorporation nevertheless makes it inaccurate to describe mother and fetus as two.[10] For the period of gestation, the fetus is wholly surrounded by and dependent upon the maternal environment. Nor is the mother independent, for she has not a moment's freedom from her responsibilities. Every action, every inaction, affects not only self but other. Whatever emotional benefits she enjoys and whatever reciprocal gifts may come later in life, at this stage the physical giving tends to be an unequal, one-way process from mother to fetus.

If the ethical category of "rights" is suited to relationships between individuals who are independent and equal, the dependence and inequality of the fetus is better represented by the ethical category of "needs." Whereas *rights* call forth corresponding *duties of respect, needs* correspond to *obligations of care.*[11-13] To sketch the broad outlines of an ethics of perinatal needs and care, we must ask who is responsible for caring for the needs of the fetus?

At first it may seem absurd to ask *who* is the ethical respondent to fetal needs. One thinks: the mother, of course. Who else? Only she is in a position, through her body, to care for the fetus. It is up to her to provide a healthful environment for fetal development through her own behavioral choices and to permit access for fetal medical or surgical interventions, if necessary.

But to limit the scope of our thinking to the immediate fetal environment is to be misled by a medical model that defines the causes of health and disease strictly in organic terms. If we adopt a broader health perspective, we will also consider a variety of contextual determinants of perinatal health. To be sure, a healthy fetus requires the support of a healthful maternal environment. Maternal health, in turn, requires a supportive and healthful family and social environment.[10,14] For example, a pregnant woman who wants to enter an inpatient treatment program for drug dependency may be able to do so only if she has a spouse or partner who can take over the family's financial obligations; if a parent, sibling or friend can care for her other young children; and if her community makes such a program accessible. A woman whose custodial work involves exposure to various chemical cleaning agents could change jobs if employers would provide for the transfer of medical and other benefits. And many women would not be smokers if their communities had prohibited the advertising of cigarettes. Perversely, in the name of free speech and the right to make a profit, we allow corporate individuals to make legal drug use attractive, then blame pregnant women for becoming addicted. *He* has a natural right to seduce; *she* has a duty to resist or suffer the consequences. Have we heard this song before?

We must, I believe, begin to think about excessive perinatal morbidity as an issue of public health and public morality and not just as an issue of individual health and morality.[15] Infant morbidity in the United States is comparatively high, yet there is no reason to think that American women are, individually, morally inferior to women in countries with healthier neonates. Rather, we have allowed our public environment to take a shape that is hostile to child health and maternal responsibility. Excessive poverty and crime, inadequate health and family services, cultural ambivalence toward drug use, obstacles to sex education, contraception and abortion—these and other features of the social environment make responsible maternity harder rather than easier. Predictably and avoidably, perinatal harms result.

If we think of the maternal-fetal dyad as the innermost nested spheres in a concentric array, this image suggests that the ethical needs at the center call forth obligations of care that ripple outward through an ethical ecosystem. In our culture of individualism, it is difficult to think of moral responsibility being spread through a system of relationships rather than as the property of an isolated individual. Nevertheless, it seems to me that exclusive reliance on the concepts of individual morality contributes to the problem of avoidable infant morbidity and cannot be expected to solve it.

Without wishing to deny that pregnant women assume serious obligations of care for meeting fetal needs, nor to deny that professional duties permit and require strong advocacy for maternal and fetal health, I do argue that medical professionals should be very cautious about acting as coercive protectors of fetal rights and enforcers of maternal duties. In most cases, this would unfairly place solely on pregnant women burdens and obligations that should be shared, complicate an already dysfunctional mother-child relationship, and discourage other women from seeking needed prenatal and perinatal care.

Greater promise rests in a more complex ethical analysis that acknowledges the mother as the focus of obligations of care for fetal needs but that also gives attention to the penumbral obligations of family and community. An ethical response to the prevalence of perinatal illness must combine clinical efforts to alter maternal behavior with attention to the mother's support systems and advocacy for policies to make the public environment more conducive to health and responsibility. The ethics of perinatal care requires a public health approach in tandem with individual interventions.

REFERENCES

1. Manning FA. Reflections on future directions of perinatal medicine. *Semin Perinatol* 1989; 13:342-51.

2. Daffos F. Access to the other patient. *Semin Perinatol* 1989; 13:252-9.

3. Beauchamp TL, McCullough LB. *Medical Ethics: The Moral Responsibilities of Physicians*. Englewood Cliffs: Prentice Hall, 1984: 27-50.

4. Chervenak FS, McCullough LB. Perinatal ethics: A practical method of analysis of obligations to mother and fetus. *Obstet Gynecol* 1985; 66:442-6.

5. DalPozzo EE, Marsh FH. Psychosis and pregnancy: Some new ethical and legal dilemmas for the physician. *Am J Obstet Gynecol* 1987; 156:425-7.

6. Robertson JA, Schulman JD. Pregnancy and prenatal harm to offspring: The case of mothers with PKU. *Hastings Center Rep* 1987; 17:23-33.

7. O'Connor DJ. *A Critical History of Western Philosophy*. New York: Free Press, 1964: 271-2.

8. Gewirth A. *Reason and Morality*. Chicago: University of Chicago Press, 1978: 135-6.

9. Englehardt HT. Current controversies in obstetrics: Wrongful life and forced fetal surgical procedures. *Am J Obstet Gynecol* 1985; 151:313-8.

10. Warren MA. Women's rights versus the protection of fetuses. *Midwest Medical Ethics* 1991; 7:1-7.

11. Gilligan C. *In A Different Voice*. Cambridge: Harvard University Press, 1982.

12. Noddings N. *Caring: A Feminine Approach to Ethics and Moral Education*. Berkeley: University of California Press, 1984.

13. Mahowald MB. *Women and Children in Health Care: An Unequal Majority*. New York: Oxford University Press, 1993.

14. Mattingly SS. The maternal-fetal dyad: Exploring the two-patient obstetric model. *Hastings Center Rep* 1992; 22:13-8.

15. Blank RH. *Mother and Fetus: Changing Notions of Maternal Responsibility*. New York: Greenwood Press, 1992: 157-71.

Cocaine:
An Overview of Use, Actions, and Effects

Shelly J. Lane

SUMMARY. The dramatic rise in cocaine use in the 1980s has prompted increased concern on the part of clinicians for both the user and, if the user is a woman of child-bearing age, for the developing fetus. The impact of prenatal cocaine exposure on the newborn has been repeatedly documented,[1-6] and plans for intervention are beginning to be developed for these newborns and their caregivers which may be of some help in getting through initial crises.[7] The long-term impact is presently poorly articulated. Although anecdotal reports of developmental concerns in prenatally exposed children at preschool and school age are available, and expectations for developmental deviations exist, research reports are not available to support these contentions. Understanding the actions of cocaine, and the implications of cocaine use, may assist parents and professionals in being realistic in both predictions and expectations. This article provides a summary of these issues. *[Article copies available from The Haworth Document Delivery Service: 1-800-342-9678. E-mail address: getinfo@haworth.com]*

BACKGROUND

Some History

Cocaine is a known stimulant, initially promoted by Sigmund Freud as a cure for many maladies, and later popularized by Sherlock Holmes.

Shelly J. Lane, PhD, OTR/L, FAOTA, is Assistant Professor, Department of Occupational Therapy, State University of New York at Buffalo, and a consultant at Children's Hospital of Buffalo, Buffalo, NY 14214-3079.

[Haworth co-indexing entry note]: "Cocaine: An Overview of Use, Actions, and Effects." Lane, Shelly J. Co-published simultaneously in *Physical & Occupational Therapy in Pediatrics* (The Haworth Press, Inc.) Vol. 16, No. 1/2, 1996, pp. 15-33; and: *Children with Prenatal Drug Exposure* (ed: Lynette S. Chandler, and Shelly J. Lane) The Haworth Press, Inc., 1996, pp. 15-33. Single or multiple copies of this article are available from The Haworth Document Delivery Service [1-800-342-9678, 9:00 a.m. - 5:00 p.m. (EST). E-mail address: getinfo@haworth.com].

© 1996 by The Haworth Press, Inc. All rights reserved.

15

Although the use of this drug has been illegal in most states since the Harrison Act of 1914-15, it has continued to be available illicitly since this time. For many years it was considered a drug of the upper and middle classes because of its high cost, but with the advent of "crack" in the early 1980's, cocaine use has increased drastically.[8]

"Crack" is a smokable form of cocaine made by mixing cocaine powder with water and baking soda which is baked to evaporate the water. Unlike cocaine powder, the chunks or "rocks" that remain following this process can be burned or smoked. The development of crack has stimulated the cocaine market because it is cheap to buy. Now easily available to all socioeconomic classes, crack has the additional attraction of not requiring the use of needles. Crack is easily absorbed through the lungs, rapidly producing a sense of intense euphoria. The euphoria is short-lived, leading to dysphoria, and often repeated use of the drug. It has been suggested that the rapid development of the crack high is behind the fact that crack is highly addictive[8,9]

The impact of the rise in cocaine use is being felt in many aspects of American life. Reports exist to document increases in crime and consequent prison overcrowding, increases in the rates of sexually transmitted diseases as users share needles or trade sexual favors for money or drugs, and, as will be seen by reading the papers in this volume, increased concern for pregnant users and the exposed fetus.[8]

Forms of Cocaine

Cocaine can be snorted (as cocaine hydrochloride), smoked (as crack), or injected (as cocaine hydrochloride mixed with water). Although snorting continues to be a common form of cocaine use, recent surveys have indicated that crack is the most commonly used form of this drug.[10] Often a new user will begin with snorting and move on to crack to achieve a more rapid and intense high. Injection of cocaine (intravenous or IV use) is more commonly seen in individuals heavily dependent on the drug, rather than in the light or casual user.[10] Cocaine concentrations in cocaine hydrochloride may vary considerably, depending upon what has been used to "cut," or dilute, the drug. Snorted cocaine is taken in "lines," which may contain as little as 3 mg, or in excess of 15 mg, of cocaine if the cocaine is at least 50% pure.[10] When crack is prepared by mixing cocaine hydrochloride with baking soda and water to form a paste, and then drying it to remove the hydrochloride,[9,11] cocaine "rocks" are produced and marketed in vials. Each vial may contain 80-100 mg of cocaine.[11] One IV "hit" typically contains 100-250 mg of cocaine, although heavy users may increase this dose to 1000 mg.[11]

Both crack and injected cocaine reach the brain within seconds, producing an almost immediate high. The crack high lasts 5-10 minutes while the injected cocaine may produce a high that lasts up to 20 minutes.[12] When snorted, the high may take several minutes to be experienced; it typically lasts 20 minutes. The high induced by cocaine is characterized by feelings of euphoria and well-being. In fact, cocaine is termed hedonic, or pleasure giving. In addition to the euphoria, crack/cocaine will instill in the user increased energy and alertness, a loss of fatigue, a feeling of enhanced physical and mental capacity, and a loss of the desire for food.[13]

Use Patterns

Cocaine use patterns differ depending on how the cocaine is taken. Crack and IV users tend to go on binges or "runs" of cocaine, during which they engage in periods of intense drug use. Binging may develop when the drug becomes more available or when larger doses are used to intensify the euphoria.[13] Binges may last for days and be followed by periods of abstinence. Cocaine binges may involve readministration of the drug as often as every 10 minutes, especially with IV use, with an average binge length of 12 hours.[13] Intravenous use of cocaine tends to lead to rapid "crashes" (within 5-15 minutes of taking the drug). A "crash" following a cocaine administration begins with mood depression, loss of energy, agitation, and intense cocaine craving.[14] These behavioral effects often lead to rapid readministration.[10,14] Individuals who snort cocaine tend to use it more often than other types of users, sometimes every day, but in lower doses.[10]

COCAINE ACTIONS

Peripheral

In the adult, cocaine is taken up into many organs, including the brain, liver, heart, and in the pregnant woman, placenta. It is rapidly broken down and essentially eliminated within 24 hours of ingestion, although urinalysis may detect cocaine or its primary metabolite, benzoylecgonine (BE), for up to three days.[10] Peripherally, cocaine produces vasoconstriction via direct action directly on the vasculature, leading to hypertension and tachycardia as a result of sympathetic nervous system activation.[10,15] In the pregnant ewe the vasoconstriction of uterine vessels has been linked to decreased uterine blood flow.[16] Plessinger and Woods have suggested that the effect of cocaine on the peripheral vasculature may be at the root of the elevated incidence of placental abruption and spontaneous abortion in pregnant human users.[15] These peripheral effects on the vasculature have been linked to inhibition of norepinephrine (NE) uptake, thereby increasing circulating (NE) levels, leading to sympathetic stimulation.[15,17]

Central

Centrally, cocaine exerts the euphoric effect described earlier via action on catecholamine and monoamine neurotransmitter systems. Increasingly, evidence from animal studies supports the hypothesis that the cocaine-induced central euphoria is mediated primarily by the mesolimbic dopamine (DA) system.[18,19] Cocaine acts on the DA neurons to increase release and inhibit reuptake of DA, thus increasing DA availability. Kuhar has suggested that the initial action of cocaine is at the DA reuptake site, and that it is here that the rewarding effects of cocaine ingestion begin.[18] Although similar uptake inhibition effects have been noted on NE neurons, central NE pathways have not been implicated in the rewarding effects of cocaine.[19] Cocaine has also been identified as a potent inhibitor of central serotonin (5HT) uptake. Because cocaine interacts with other aspects of this system, it has been suggested that 5HT plays at least a secondary role in the central euphoric effects of cocaine.[20] Moreover, Gawin and Kleber have hypothesized that the rewarding influence and euphoria induced by cocaine may be caused by an interaction between the 5HT and the catecholamine systems (DA and NE).[21] Further investigation into this possibility is warranted.

Medical complications associated with cocaine use include heart attacks, cerebral hemorrhage, heatstroke, seizures, respiratory failure, chronic nasal problems, and lung and heart damage.[10] Cocaine overdose can result in death. Other complications associated with cocaine use are related to the substances with which the cocaine has been "cut" and to IV use. Commonly used cutting substances include ammonia, starch and talc. The latter two cutting substances are hypothesized to lead to chronic lung inflammation secondary to obstruction of small blood vessels. Intravenous use is associated with an increased incidence of skin and deep tissue infection at the sight of injection. In addition, IV users may develop endocarditis as a result of bacteria introduced into the circulation. Because IV users often share needles, hepatitis is commonly found. Finally, exposure to HIV and the subsequent development of AIDS form a critical, and at present eventually fatal, complication of IV drug use.[10]

Long-Term Use and Withdrawal. Long-term use of cocaine has been shown by some investigators to lead to sustained neurophysiologic changes in central neurotransmitter systems, especially those associated with mood and the experience of pleasure.[13] It has been hypothesized that long-term use leads to specific changes in neurotransmitter system function in the brain, and that withdrawal subsequently results in supersensitivity of the DA receptors which regulate DA release.[14] This leads to decreased release of DA, which produces the anhedonia associated with withdrawal in humans.[13] Characteristics of "cocaine withdrawal" have been described by Gawin and his colleagues.[13,14,21] They delineated a sequence of events beginning with Phase 1, defined as the crash following a binge. This crash results from exhausting the available supply of cocaine and being unable to obtain more, or from an acute tolerance to the euphoric effects of cocaine, despite increased doses. As noted earlier, it includes depression, irritability, anxiety, confusion, insomnia, and a gradually diminishing craving for the drug.[10,21] Withdrawal is also associated with decreased energy, limited interest in the environment, and increased need for sleep.[13,21] Phase 1 symptoms may intensify over 12-96 hours following abstinence.

Phase 2 is characterized by initial mood functioning that approaches normal, followed by substantial anhedonia, anxiety, irritability, lack of energy, and continued cocaine craving. Cocaine craving is triggered by environmental cues, e.g., seeing old friends with whom the individual used to use cocaine. These characteristics often lead to a subsequent binge. Phase 1 and 2 may cycle repeatedly in individuals who abuse cocaine. Gawin and Kleber report that this pattern of binging, crashing, having a few days of near normal function (during which time many individuals may feel they have control over the drug), increased craving, and binging again, may repeat for many months.[21]

Phase 3 is described by Gawin and Kleber as the phase of "extinction."[21] If an individual has broken the cycle described above, the extinction phase will develop. It is characterized by a return to a more normal mood state, but with continued craving for cocaine. The cravings during this phase are reported to be less severe, but they may be present for months or years after an individual has been abstinent.[13] Maintained abstinence from cocaine reduces the intensity of the craving. Because craving is triggered by environmental cues, inpatient intervention for cocaine dependence may be ineffective because the inpatient avoids environmental triggers which s/he will face again once they are "outside" the treatment center.[13]

INVESTIGATING PRENATAL IMPACT

The Study of Prenatal Exposure

The study of cocaine effects on the fetus is fraught with problems. Individuals using cocaine rarely use this drug alone; commonly it is used in conjunction with amphetamines, marijuana, alcohol, tobacco, and caffeine.[9,22] Because each of these substances has been shown to have its own effect on the developing fetus, attributing developmental deviations or deficits to cocaine becomes tenuous and dependent upon the researcher's ability to control for confounding factors. In addition, in adult users it is often difficult to establish the frequency of use, as well as the dose. As noted earlier, different use patterns exist and these are likely to exert different effects on the developing fetus.

Drug use history is difficult to establish because self-report of drug use has questionable reliability and validity. Under-reporting by pregnant women, and the population of cocaine users as a whole, is common because of the potential ramifications of accurate portrayals of use.[23,24] Even in cases in which the mother is willing to reveal frequency and dose of the drug, the purity of the drug is often in question, thus making "dose" a relative term.[12] Given the likelihood that exposure to cocaine will result in different effects depending upon timing during gestation, exposure dose, and exposure frequency, the lack of accurate reporting presents a considerable hurdle to understanding the effects of cocaine exposure in utero.

Detection of Maternal Use

Because of the unreliability of maternal self-report of drug use, few investigators of drug effects rely solely on this method.[25] Analytic methods currently in use include urinalysis, and meconium and hair analysis. Some investigators recommend that self-report be used in addition to chemical analysis for a more complete picture of drug use throughout pregnancy.[25] Each analysis method will be addressed below.

The most frequently reported means of detecting neonatal cocaine exposure is urine toxicology screening administered at birth. This procedure requires urine collection as soon as possible following birth and detects cocaine exposure (by detecting both cocaine and BE in the urine) for between 3-5 days before testing.[24] Thus, one shortcoming of urine screening is that it provides information about cocaine use only for the very recent past. Drug use early in pregnancy, or even in the later stages of pregnancy but not immediately prior to delivery, is not detectable by this method. Interestingly, this same shortcoming has been noted to be a strength in that other detection techniques *cannot* detect cocaine use in the immediate past.[26] Urinalysis utilizes an arbitrary cutoff level, and as such, when amounts of cocaine or BE detected are below the cutoff, a negative result is reported.[27] As a result, there is a high false negative report rate; urine screening may miss 50% or more of prenatal exposure cases when compared to a newer and promising method, meconium analysis.[28]

Analysis of meconium requires the collection of the baby's first stool (meconium) during the first few days post-birth. Meconium is a waste product normally excreted by the newborn after birth. Because it is accumulated throughout gestation, it offers a view of drug exposure that extends beyond the days immediately prior to birth.[28] Meconium analysis can detect cocaine as well as other substances of abuse (e.g., opiates and cannabinoids) with greater sensitivity and specificity than urinalysis.[28] A cut-off level has been established by one group of investigators to represent "background" readings for normal meconium;[28] it is lower than the cut-off referred to above for urinalysis.[29] In addition to the improved detection rate shown with meconium analysis, it is four times more accurate in detecting recent drug use than self-report.[28] Ostrea and colleagues report that this technique lends itself well to use in typical clinical laboratories and that it can be modified for automated analysis.[29] Meconium analysis is still under investigation and not widely used at present; however, it holds much promise for the future.

Hair analysis is another alternative detection method under investigation. This technique detects cocaine metabolites in adult users and infants and can detect prior exposure even when urinalysis results are negative. Graham and colleagues[30] recommend using hair analysis in conjunction with urine analysis because hair analysis cannot detect use in the immediate past. Instead, because of the deposition of BE on the hair shaft, hair analysis can detect long term cocaine use.[27,30] Furthermore, hair analysis has the potential to distinguish periods of use from periods of no-use, based on the concentration of drug metabolite found in different locations on the hair shaft. This has important implications because self-reported drug use histories have been established to be less than adequate in providing an accurate picture of prior patterns of drug use.[27] In spite of these seemingly positive characteristics, hair analysis has not been completely embraced. Even proponents of this technique admit that it is an expensive process.[31] In addition, the amount of hair required for analysis may be prohibitive, especially if the subject for study is a newborn.[26] Furthermore, the ability of these analyses to distinguish between passive exposure and actual drug use has been questioned. Passive exposure to illicit drugs can result in deposition on the hair shaft, although the concentration of drugs in this instance is much lower[27] and, while cocaine itself is deposited, BE is not.[32] Furthermore, investigators supporting use of hair analysis have shown that proper preparation of the hair before analysis will remove substances deposited in this manner.[27,32] Additional criticism, however, comes from an absence of standardization in the process of preparing hair for analysis, leading to differences in findings from one lab to another.[27] Nonetheless, some investigators favor this technique over urinalysis. Mieczkowski and colleagues note that hair analysis has advantages over urinalysis in that samples are highly stable, they can more readily be collected, abstinence for several days prior to testing will not lead to negative test results, and "flushing" by drinking large quantities of water just prior to sample collection is not possible.[31] Further investigation and fine tuning of analysis methods has been recommended.[27]

Animal Models for Investigation of Prenatal Effects

Animal models of substance use have been developed to circumvent some of the shortcomings of human research and to further our understanding of in utero drug effects. In these studies substance type, use pattern, and dose can be controlled. A substantial foundation of information has been developed based on animal models of human substance use. This information base has guided research on infants and children, but it must be kept in mind that making the jump from animal to human research has its own perils. For instance, fetal growth inhibition was detected in early prenatal cocaine exposure studies in rats.[33] This finding correlates well with the low birth weight noted in the human infant following prenatal cocaine exposure.[3,6,34,35] In rats, however, the level of cocaine exposure needed to induce growth inhibition greatly exceeds the levels found in humans using cocaine recreationally.[24] Thus, the relationship between these human and rat findings is unclear. In addition, there are substantial differences in gestation between rat and human: the final trimester of development in the human is comparable to early extrauterine development in the rat. Other animal models, such as the pregnant ewe or primate, provide a closer, but still somewhat tenuous, link. In addition, the complex lifestyles of humans, particularly those using illicit drugs, play a role in both prenatal and postnatal development that cannot be duplicated in animal studies.[23,24] According to Dow-Edwards,[24, p.348] "cocaine use is part of a lifestyle which includes poverty, poly-drug abuse, poor health, STD and human immunodeficiency virus (HIV)." Thus, although we must look to research on animal models for information and guidance, it is wise to use caution when applying these findings to human infants and children.

COCAINE EFFECTS ON THE FETUS

Cocaine and the Placenta

As a highly water- and lipid-soluble substance with low molecular weight, cocaine passes through both the blood-brain barrier and the placental barrier with little resistance. In doing so, cocaine can produce direct effects on the fetus.[36] In pregnant rats a single dose of cocaine was found to reach maximal concentrations in the fetal brain by approximately 30 minutes following exposure.[37] In addition, although cocaine is found in many fetal tissues, it has been shown to concentrate in fetal rat brain as the result of an ineffective blood-brain barrier.[38] Reports of fetal brain concentrations vary. One investigation demonstrated greater fetal than maternal rat brain concentrations of cocaine,[37] while other studies have shown lower fetal levels in rat, mouse, and ewe.[39-41] An investigation using monkeys indicated that, from a single dose of cocaine administered in a quantity comparable to a snorted dose of 0.10 gms, 30% crossed the placental barrier and entered the fetal circulation within 30-60 minutes of ingestion.[42] Levels of BE were demonstrated to be higher in the fetal rat brain than the adult rat brain by Spear and colleagues.[41] This finding is of great interest because BE is an *active* cocaine metabolite, i.e., in the adult BE has been shown to have stimulatory effects. The investigators suggest that high levels of BE in the fetal rat brain tissue may have an adverse impact on the developing brain.[41] Clearance of cocaine from fetal rat tissue is not as effective as in the adult because of immaturity of enzymes that degrade cocaine.[36] As a result, exposure to the drug may be prolonged. An interesting investigation using human placentas indicated that, in the later part of a term pregnancy, the placenta may provide protection from cocaine, in that it can metabolize cocaine into less active by-products.[17] Unfortunately for the fetus, such protection is not present in the first trimester when animal studies indicate easy passage of both cocaine and BE across the placenta and into the developing brain. If these studies can be extrapolated to humans, there is cause for concern. Coupling this information with the reported patterns of use in humans suggests that some exposed infants may experience repeated high doses of cocaine at vulnerable periods in development. Other fetuses may experience continual low doses of cocaine throughout pregnancy. The different effects of such diverse exposure have not been elucidated, and the possibility that they exist impairs our ability to offer general statements about what to expect from babies who have experienced prenatal cocaine exposure.

Cocaine and the Fetus

Fetal effects of in utero cocaine exposure may be both direct and indirect. Direct effects are those mediated by the cocaine as it acts on the fetal brain, circulation, and so on. Some of these effects are similar to those noted above for the adult, while others may differ as a result of the immaturity of the fetal system. Indirect effects associated with prenatal cocaine exposure are those that follow from cocaine use by the mother. Maternal malnutrition, which results in malnutrition for the fetus, is one example of such an indirect effect. Prenatal undernutrition alone has been associated with lower birth weight. Direct and indirect effects are described separately in the following sections.

Direct Effects. In the fetus, as in the mother, cocaine induces both peripheral and central vasoconstriction[16] which has been associated with the development of cardiovascular, genitourinary, gastrointestinal, and musculoskeletal anomalies.[17] In addition, the growth retardation associated with cocaine exposure has been linked to fetal vasoconstriction by some investigators.[35] Vasoconstriction can lead to hypoxia which results in a release of catecholamines. It has been suggested that cocaine may also interact with catecholamine systems in the fetus, much like effects in the mother.[17] Thus, acutely, cocaine increases catecholamine release and blocks reuptake. Animal literature suggests that long-term use of cocaine produces an attenuation of dopaminergic function in rats,[43] and that the changes in the DA system can be correlated with changes in glucose utilization.[44] In a related human study Needlman and colleagues[45] presented preliminary results indicating lower levels of homovanillic acid (HVA) in the cerebrospinal fluid of neonates exposed prenatally to cocaine (and other substances). The decrease in this metabolite of DA may reflect reduced DA production or DA depletion. Although the sample size in the study was small, the difference persisted when investigators controlled for confounding variables such as cigarette smoking, alcohol use, and use of other drugs. Although this finding requires further substantiation, it coincides with indications of reduced DA function in cocaine-exposed animals and suggests that newborns may experience attenuated function in at least the DA system. Mirochnick and colleagues[46] also reported increased circulating levels of dihydroxyphenylalanine (DOPA) in cocaine-exposed newborns. DOPA is a precursor to both NE and DA. Increased levels of this precursor may indicate that less is being used to produce DA, further substantiating the possibility of reduced DA production in newborns following prenatal cocaine exposure. In this same work, a trend toward increased NE levels was also found. Of interest was their finding that NE levels had an inverse relationship with Neonatal Behavior Assessment Scale performance on the test's orientation cluster: increased NE levels were associated with decreased auditory and visual responsiveness. Thus, the direct effect of cocaine on the fetal catecholamine systems has the potential to adversely affect sensory function after birth.

Both DA and 5HT may play a role in behavioral regulation. The depletion of DA, which may parallel the lower HVA levels, may be related to the difficulty of cocaine-exposed neonates to demonstrate state modulation.[47] Prenatal exposure to cocaine in rats has also been associated with changes in 5HT in the early postnatal period. Akbari and colleagues[48] reported delayed growth of 5HT fibers to the cortex and hippocampus in rats. This structural deviation is no longer present at four postnatal weeks. Because we know that DA plays a role in activity level and attention, as well as in motor control, and that 5HT has been associated with attention, it is easy to jump to the conclusion that early cocaine-induced changes in the dopaminergic and serotonergic systems provide a causal link with the behavioral problems and perhaps with motor deficits noted in human infants following such prenatal exposure. As noted earlier, differences between rats and humans are large, and these conclusions have yet to be substantiated. It is critical to keep in mind that the type and severity of any teratologic effects of cocaine are related to the timing of use, the dose, and its frequency.[15]

Indirect Effects. Indirect effects of cocaine on the developing fetus stem from the direct effects the drug has on the mother. As noted earlier, in pregnancy cocaine causes increased maternal blood pressure and placental vasoconstriction by inhibiting the reuptake of norepinephrine at neurons innervating the vasculature. The result is uteroplacental insufficiency which alone has been correlated with low birth weight and growth retardation as well as tachycardia.[17,23] In addition to the insufficiency, vasoconstriction can lead to fetal hypoxia.[16]

Beyond these physiologic effects, cocaine also reduces maternal appetite.[10] Although not a universal finding, decreased weight gain in pregnant users has been reported.[6,49] Frank and colleagues state that even beyond appetite reduction, cocaine may impair the transfer of nutrients from mother to fetus as a result of uterine vessel vasoconstriction.[50] In contrast, Dicke and colleagues[51] have recently shown that cocaine can interfere with the transport of alanine, an amino acid needed for fetal growth, from maternal to fetal plasma. These authors suggested that maternal and fetal vasoconstriction may not be sufficient to impair fetal growth because it is relatively short-lived. They offer an alternative interpretation: cocaine interferes with the transport of critical nutrients, such as alanine, leading to inadequate growth and development. It has also been hypothesized that the increase in fetal metabolism, directly induced by fetal cocaine exposure, may deplete stores of nutrients in the fetus, resulting in malnutrition and subsequent low birth weight.[50] Thus, the growth retardation that has been associated with prenatal cocaine use may be related to several factors. Finally, research suggests that babies born with low birth weight are at greater risk than others for the development of later, perhaps subtle, problems with both behavior and learning.[52]

Fathers' Contribution to Prenatal Exposure

Recent investigations indicate that there may be another avenue by which the fetus can be exposed to drugs in utero. Cocaine has been shown to bind to sperm cells. Yazigi and colleagues[53] reported that cocaine will bind to human spermatozoa and that such binding does not impair the sperm cell motility or viability. In addition, an examination of the distribution of cocaine within genital organs in mice indicated that, of all organs tested, cocaine concentrations were highest in the kidney and epididymis.[54] These authors suggested that these findings may explain the teratogenesis noted in some cases when maternal cocaine use is both denied and cannot be identified with current analytic tools.

IMPACT OF SUBSTANCE ABUSE
ON THE MOTHER/INFANT RELATIONSHIP

Investigations of substance abuse have not typically focused on women, however, a growing body of information addresses the impact on mother/infant interaction and/or bonding. Although some of this literature is specific to the impact of cocaine, the bulk of the research is with mothers using opioids or a combination of illicit substances. The information presented next is drawn from this heterogeneous body of literature and, when it applies specifically to cocaine, this will be noted.

Studies examining prevalence of use in women have largely focused on inner city minority populations. Although actual percentages vary even in this select group of women, statistics indicate that 10 to 20% of women, and sometimes more, have used cocaine at least once during their pregnancies.[25,55,56] Frank and colleagues reported that nearly half of their primarily non-white, urban population reported use of cocaine during only one trimester of pregnancy; 18% reported using the drug throughout gestation.[25] When private pay and public health clinic patients are examined separately, prevalence of use during pregnancy varies. Chasnoff and colleagues examined urine samples during a one-month time frame from all pregnant women enrolling in prenatal care in both environments. These investigators found a nearly equivalent rate between the two groups (13.1 and 16.3%, respectively).[57] In contrast, Matera and colleagues collected urine from all women delivering in a New York City hospital over a 6 week period of time. The results of this investigation indicated that 14% of health clinic patients, compared to 1.4% of private patients, tested positive for cocaine at the time of delivery.[55] Schutzman and associates used meconium analysis to examine prevalence in a suburban hospital setting and reported that 6.3% of private pay and 26.9% of Medicaid or uninsured babies tested positive for cocaine exposure.[56] To complicate the matter both for the child and for mother-child relationships, numerous investigations indicate that cocaine use is often accompanied by use of other illicit substances.[23,25,55,56]

Although these prevalence rates are striking, alone they do not address the issue of mother/child relationships. It has been suggested that "the highly addictive qualities of cocaine often reduce the likelihood that mothers will seek prenatal care, or increase the probability that they will postpone initiation of prenatal care until late in the pregnancy."[58, p.34] The mothering role then is poorly assumed from the outset of pregnancy. What is the impact of continued maternal drug use on the ability to nurture and care for children? The answer to this question is complex.

The mother who continues to use substances has a greater propensity for poor caregiving for a variety of reasons. Appropriate social support systems for these mothers are limited, as are intervention systems.[59] It has been suggested that the majority of women using illicit substances have histories of abuse and neglect as both adults and children.[25] They may have never experienced nurturing themselves, resulting in a failure to provide the warmth and nurturance needed to form a solid parent/child bond with their own child.[60] Such mothers are at greater risk for development of both physical and mental illness that may reduce their ability to care for themselves and their families.[61] Continued drug use can diminish the motivation to care for infant and family, placing the infant at risk for abuse or neglect or both.[61] Furthermore, the lifestyle of mothers who continue to use illicit substances is not conducive to adequate caregiving. Instead, this lifestyle places the infant at risk for the secondary consequences of violent crime and passive exposure to drugs in the home.[60] Of interest is that exposure to cocaine beyond the prenatal period has been linked with seizures in infants and preadolescent children.[61] Likely routes of exposure in these cases included accidental oral ingestion, passive inhalation, and second-hand smoke inhalation.[61-65] Such cocaine-related seizures are most often single events with no long lasting sequelae,[61-64] although some incidents of on-going seizure disorder are reported.[61] Although the exact relationship between seizures and cocaine exposure in the young child is not clear, in at least some cases the seizures are associated with infantile fever.[61]

Establishment of the mother/infant relationship is an integral component of the mothering role, and the interaction between mother and child influences the infant's capacity for future positive social-emotional and intellectual development.[66-68] Mothers who use illicit substances and quit, have the potential to form secure, supportive attachments with their children.[69] Rodnig and colleagues[70] indicate that it is the continued use of drugs that interferes with parenting ability and places the mother/child relationship at risk. Maternal conditions associated with continued drug dependency may affect the mother's ability to behave in the consistent, responsible manner needed to initiate a successful nurturing relationship with her infant.[71] In this mother-infant dyad the cocaine-using mother has been noted to be less proficient in maintaining interaction with her infant because of difficulty reading and responding appropriately to infant cues.[58,59] A small study of cocaine- and polydrug-using mothers indicated that the social initiative and resourcefulness with infants demonstrated by this group of mothers were seriously compromised, leading to infants who did not show typical happiness.[22] The interaction pattern between mother and child was one with a minimum of enthusiasm and enjoyment. Mothers in this study were also identified as lacking flexibility and as providing minimal structure for the infant.[22] Other studies have shown that substance-using mothers may detach themselves from the infant or approach the infant in a flat, unresponsive manner.[71] Furthermore, these mothers often have unrealistic expectations regarding their child's potential and skills.[71] The combination of inadequate mothering and an irritable baby may result in a severely compromised mother-infant relationship. In addition to these issues, mothers using cocaine may have ongoing feelings of guilt and concerns about their own ability to cope and meet the demands of the infant.[72] Thus, for mothers who continue to use illicit drugs after the birth of their child, the occupational role of "mother" is inadequately expressed.

LONG-TERM EFFECTS ON BEHAVIOR

Follow-up into adulthood of rats exposed to cocaine prenatally points to continued deficits. Rat studies have shown that the hippocampus is functionally depressed in adults that were prenatally exposed to cocaine.[73] Memory and learning in these animals are impaired.[48] In addition, persistent deficits in function of the nigrostriatal pathway (fine motor coordination) have also been noted.[73] This and other work of Dow-Edwards is strongly suggestive of long-term alterations in central dopamine function in rats following prenatal cocaine exposure.[24]

Understanding long-term outcome for human infants is just beginning. Human outcome studies will not be reviewed here because this information is included in the current volume both as reports of recent research and as reviews. Bayer and colleagues present short-term effects relative to visual retention memory; Giusti addresses development at 12-28 months, as determined by the Battelle Developmental Inventory; Swanson, and Arendt, Minnes, and Singer review neuromotor, cognitive and behavioral outcomes; the latter authors also present a summary of their developmental findings in infants at 17 months of age. Even given this amount of information, it is not clear how these children will deal with the stresses of school, adolescence, or adulthood. Although some initial reports stated that children prenatally exposed to cocaine were more withdrawn or difficult to control in classroom settings, that the children would experience difficulty adapting to a typical school environment,[74] and that these children formed a "bio-underclass" who would require special education,[75] these concerns have not been borne out with further research. We must await the results of careful, long-term studies in order to develop an accurate picture of the outcomes of prenatal cocaine-exposure in the human infant.

CONCLUSION

Great potential exists for the development of problems following prenatal cocaine exposure. Evidence is mounting to substantiate developmental deviations during the neonatal and early infancy period in humans. Furthermore, such exposure certainly places children at *high risk* for later problems. It is imperative, however, that we remain unbiased in assessing these children as they grow. Although speculation and the popular press may tell us that there are devastating long-term effects of prenatal cocaine exposure, at present we do not have the research to support these statements. Greer, an educator, has labeled these children "neurochemical timebombs."[75] Put simply, we need more information before such a global statement can be made with confidence.

REFERENCES

1. Chasnoff IJ, Lewis DE, Griffith DR, Willey S. Cocaine and pregnancy: Clinical and toxicological implications for the neonate. *Clin Chem.* 1989;35:1276-1278.

2. Cohen ME, Anday EK, Kelley NE, Hoffman HS. Sensorineural reactivity as assessed by reflex modification in neonates following intrauterine exposure to cocaine. *Pediatr Res.* 1988(4pt2);23:209A. Abstract.

3. Frank DA, Bauchner H, Parker S, Huber A, Kyel-Aboagye K, Cabral H, Zuckerman B. Neonatal body proportionality and body composition after in utero exposure to cocaine and marijuana. *J Pediatr.* 1990;117:622-626.

4. Mayes LC, Granger RH, Frank MA, Schottenfeld R, Bornstein MH. Neurobehavioral profiles of neonates exposed to cocaine prenatally. *Pediatrics.* 1993;91:778-783.

5. Schneider JW, Chasnoff IJ. Cocaine abuse during pregnancy: Its effects on infant motor development–A clinical perspective. *Top Acute Care Trauma Rehabil.* 1987;2:59-69.

6. Zuckerman B, Frank D, Hingson R, Amaro H, Levenson SM, Kayne H, Parker S, Vinci R, Aboagye K, Fried LE, Cabral H, Timperi R, Bouchner H. Effects of maternal marijuana and cocaine on fetal growth. *N Engl J Med.* 1989;320:762-768.

7. Schneider JW, Griffith DR, Chasnoff IJ. Infants exposed to cocaine in utero: Implications for developmental assessment and intervention. *Inf Young Child.* 1989;2:25-36.

8. Kandall SR. Perinatal effects of cocaine and amphetamine use during pregnancy. *Bull NY Acad Sci.* 1991;67:240-255.

9. Smart RG. Crack cocaine use: A review of prevalence and adverse effects. *Am J Drug Alcohol Abuse.* 1991;17:13-26.

10. Weiss RD, Mirin SM, Bartel RL eds. *Cocaine Second Edition.* Washington DC: American Psychiatric Press, Inc.; 1994:27-49.

11. Belenko SR. *Crack and the Evolution of Anti-Drug Policy.* Westport, CT: Greenwood Press; 1993.

12. Pottieger AE, Tressel PA, Inciardi JA, Rosales TA. Cocaine use patterns and overdose. *J Psychoactive Drugs.* 1992;24:399-410.

13. Gawin FH, Ellingwood EH. Cocaine and other stimulants–actions, abuse, and treatment. *N Engl J Med.* 1988;318:1173-1182.

14. Gawin FH. Cocaine addiction: Psychology and neurophysiology. *Science.* 1991;251:1580-1586.

15. Plessinger MA, Woods JR. The cardiovascular effects of cocaine use in pregnancy. *Reprod Toxicol.* 1991;5:99-113.

16. Woods JR, Plessinger MA, Clark EI. Effect of cocaine on uterine blood flow and fetal oxygenation. *JAMA.* 1987;257:957-961.

17. Roe DA, Little BB, Bawdon RE, Gilstrap LC. Metabolism of cocaine by human placentas: Implications for fetal exposure. *Am J Obstet Gynecol.* 1990;163:715-718.

18. Kuhar MJ. Molecular pharmacology of cocaine: A dopamine hypothesis and its implications. In: Bock GR, Whelan J eds. *Cocaine: Scientific and Social Dimensions.* New York: John Wiley & Sons; 1992:81-95.

19. Fibiger HC, Phillips AG, Brown EE. The neurobiology of cocaine-induced reinforcement. In: Bock GR, Whelan J eds. *Cocaine: Scientific and Social Dimensions.* New York: John Wiley & Sons; 1992:96-111.

20. Wolf WA, Kuhn DM. Cocaine and serotonin neurochemistry. *Neurochem Int.* 1991;18:33-38.

21. Gawin FH, Kleber HD. Abstinence symptomatology and psychiatric diagnosis in cocaine abusers. *Arch Gen Psychiatry.* 1986;43:107-113.

22. Burns K, Chethik L, Burns WJ, Clark R. Dyadic disturbances in cocaine-abusing mothers and their infants. *J Clin Psychol.* 1991;47:316-319.

23. MacGregor SN, Keith LG, Chasnoff IJ, Rosner MA, Chisum GM, Shaw P, Minogue JP. Cocaine use during pregnancy: Adverse perinatal outcome. *Am J Obstet Gynecol.* 1987;157:686-690.

24. Dow-Edwards DL. Cocaine effects on fetal development: A comparison of clinical and animal research findings. *Neurotoxicol Teratol.* 1991;13:347-352.

25. Frank DA, Zuckerman BS, Amaro H, Aboagye K, Bauchner H, Cabral H, Fried L, Hingson R, Kayne H, Levenson SM, Parker S, Reece H, Vinci R. Cocaine use during pregnancy: Prevalence and correlates. *Pediatrics.* 1988;82:888-895.

26. Bailey DN. Drug screening in an unconventional matrix: Hair analysis. *JAMA.* 1989;262:3331.

27. Mieczkowski T. New approaches in drug testing: A review of hair analysis. *Ann Am Acad Pol Soc Sci.* 1992;521:132-150.

28. Ostrea EM, Brady M, Gause S, Raymundo AL, Stevens M. Drug screening of newborns by meconium analysis: A large-scale, prospective epidemiologic study. *Pediatrics.* 1992;89:107-113.

29. Ostrea EM, Romero AI, Yee H. Adaptation of the meconium drug test for mass screening. *J Pediatr.* 1993;122:152-154.

30. Graham K, Koren G, Klein J, Schneiderman J, Greenwald M. Determination of gestational cocaine exposure by hair analysis. *JAMA.* 1989;262:3328-3330.

31. Mieczkowski T, Barzelay D, Gropper B, Wish E. Concordance of three measures of cocaine use in an arrestee population: Hair, urine, and self-report. *J Psychoact Drugs.* 1991;23:241-249.

32. Koren G, Klein J, Forman R, Graham K. Hair analysis of cocaine: Differentiation between systemic exposure and external contamination. *J Clin Pharmacol.* 1992;32: 671-675.

33. Church, MW, Pintcheff BF, Gessner PK. Dose-dependent consequences of cocaine in pregnancy outcome in the Long-Evans rat. *Neurotoxicol Teratol.* 1988;10:51-58.

34. Chasnoff IJ, Burns WJ, Schnoll SH, Burns KA. Cocaine use in pregnancy. *N Engl J Med.* 1985;313:666-669.

35. Cherukuri R, Minkoff H, Feldman J, Parekh A, Glass L. A cohort study of alkaloidal cocaine ("crack") in pregnancy. *Obstet Gynecol.* 1988;72:147-151.

36. Dow-Edwards D. Fetal and maternal cocaine levels peak rapidly following intragastric administration in the rat. *J Subst Abuse.* 1990;2:427-437.

37. DeVane CL, Simpkins JW, Miller RL, Braun SB. Tissue distribution of cocaine in the pregnant rat. *Life Sci.* 1989;45:1271-1276.

38. Wiggins RC. Pharmacokinetics of cocaine in pregnancy and effects on fetal maturation. *Clin Pharmacokinet.* 1992;22:85-93.

39. Moore TR, Sorg J, Miller L, Key TC, Resnick R. Hemodynamic effects of intravenous cocaine on the pregnant ewe and fetus. *Am J Obstet Gynecol.* 1986;155: 883-888.

40. Shah NS, May DA, Yates JD. Disposition of levo-[^{3}H]cocaine in pregnant and nonpregnant mice. *Toxicol Appl Pharmacol.* 1980;53: 279-284.

41. Spear LP, Kirstein CL, Frambes NA. Cocaine effects on the developing central nervous system: Behavioral, psychopharmacological, and neurochemical studies. *Ann NY Acad Sci.* 1989;562:290-307.

42. Fackelmann KA. The maternal cocaine connection. *Sci News.* 1991;140: 152-153.

43. Spear LP, Frambes N, Kirstein CL, Bell J, Rogers L, Youttanasumpun V, Spear NE. Neurobehavioral teratogenic effects of prenatal exposure to cocaine. *Behav Teratol Soc Abstracts.* 1988;37:518.

44. Dow-Edwards DL, Fico T, Hutchings DE. Functional effects of cocaine given during critical periods of development. *Behav Teratol Soc Abstracts.* 1988;37:518.

45. Needlman R, Zuckerman B, Anderson GM, Micochnick M, Cohen DJ. Cerebrospinal fluid monoamine precursors and metabolites in human neonates following in utero cocaine exposure: A preliminary study. *Pediatrics.* 1993;92:55-60.

46. Mirochnick M, Meyer J, Cole J, Herren T, Zuckerman B. Circulating catecholamine concentrations in cocaine-exposed neonates: A pilot study. *Pediatrics.* 1991;88:481-485.

47. Zuckerman B, Bresnahan K. Developmental and behavioral consequences of prenatal drug and alcohol exposure. *Pediatr Clin North Am.* 1991;38:1387-1406.

48. Akbari HM, Kramer HK, Whitaker-Azmitia PM, Spear LP, Azmitia EC. Prenatal cocaine exposure disrupts the development of the serotonergic system. *Brain Res.* 1992;572:57-63.

49. Petiti DB, Cleman C. Cocaine and the risk of low birth weight. *Am J Public Health.* 1990;80:25-28.

50. Frank DA, Bresnahan K, Zuckerman BS. Maternal cocaine use: Impact on child health and development. *Adv Pediatr.* 1993;40:65-99.

51. Dicke JM, Verges DK, Polakoski KL. Cocaine inhibits alanine uptake by human placental microvillous membrane vesicles. *Am J Obstet Gynecol.* 1993;169:515-521.

52. Tomchek S, Lane SJ. Full-term low birth weight infants: Etiology and implications for development. *Phys Occup Ther Pediatr.* 1994;13(3):43-46.

53. Yazigi RA, Odem RR, Polakoski KL. Demonstration of specific binding of cocaine to human spermatozoa. *JAMA.* 1991;266:1956-1959.

54. Yazigi RA, Polakoski KL. Distribution of tritiated cocaine in selected genital and nongenital organs following administration to male mice. *Arch Pathol Lab Med.* 1992;116:1036-1039.

55. Matera C, Warren WB, Moomjy M, Fink DJ, Fox HE. Prevalence of use of cocaine and other substances in an obstetric population. *Am J Obstet Gynecol.* 1990;163:797-801.

56. Schutzman DL, Frankenfield-Chernicoff M, Clatterbaugh HE, Singer J. Incidence of intrauterine cocaine exposure in a suburban setting. *Pediatrics.* 1991;88:825-827.

57. Chasnoff IJ, Landress HJ, Barrett ME. The prevalence of illicit-drug or alcohol use during pregnancy and discrepancies in mandatory reporting in Pinellas County, Florida. *N Engl J Med.* 1990;322:1202-1206.
58. Thurman SK, Berry BE. Cocaine use: Implications for intervention with childbearing women and their infants. *Children's Health Care.* 1992;21:31-38.
59. Bresnahan K, Brooks C, Zuckerman B. Prenatal cocaine use: Impact on infants and mothers. *Pediatr Nurs.* 1991;17:123-129.
60. Kronstadt D. Complex developmental issues of prenatal drug exposure. *Future of Children.* 1991;1:36-49.
61. Mott SH, Packer RJ, Soldin AJ. Neurologic manifestations of cocaine exposure in childhood. *Pediatr.* 1994;93:557-560.
62. Rivikin M, Gilmore HE. Generalized seizures in an infant due to environmentally acquired cocaine. *Pediatr.* 1989;84:1100-1102.
63. Ernst AA, Sanders WM. Unexpected cocaine intoxication presenting as seizures in children. *Ann Emerg Med.* 1989;18:774-777.
64. Bateman DA, Heagarty MC. Passive freebase cocaine ('Crack') inhalation by infants and toddlers. *AJDC.* 1989;143:25-27.
65. Dinnies JD, Darr CD, Saulys AJ. Cocaine toxicity in toddlers. *AJDC.* 1990;144:743-744.
66. Haskett ME, Miller WJ, Whitworth JM, Huffman JM. Intervention with cocaine-abusing mothers. *J Contemp Human Serv.* 1992;Oct.:451-462.
67. Blehar MC, Lieberman AF, Ainsworth MD. Early face to face interaction and its relation to later infant-mother attachment. *Child Dev.* 1977;48:182-194.
68. Lewis M, Coates DL. Mother-infant interaction and cognitive development in twelve week old infants. *Inf Beh Dev.* 1980;3:95-105.
69. Mahoney G, Powell A. Modifying parent-child interaction: Enhancing the development of handicapped children. *J Spec Ed.* 1988;22:82-96.
70. Rodning C, Beckwith L, Howard J. Quality of attachment and home environments in children prenatally exposed to PCP and cocaine. *Dev Psychopathol.* 1991;3:351-366.
71. Lief NR. The drug user as a parent. *Int J Addict.* 1985;20:63-97.
72. Griffith DR. The effects of perinatal cocaine exposure on infant neurobehavior and early maternal-infant interactions. In: Chasnoff IJ ed. *Drugs, Alcohol, Pregnancy and Parenting.* Dordrecht, Germany: Kluwer Academic Publishers; 1988:105-113.
73. Dow-Edwards DL, Freed LA, Fico TA. Structural and functional effects of prenatal cocaine exposure in adult rat brain. *Dev Brain Res.* 1990;57:263-268.
74. Rist MC. The shadow children. *School Board J.* 1990; Jan:19-24.
75. Greer JV. The drug babies. *Excep Child.* 1990;56:382-384.

Neuromotor Outcome of Infants Exposed Prenatally to Cocaine: Issues of Assessment and Interpretation

Marcia W. Swanson

SUMMARY. The effect of prenatal cocaine exposure on the neuromotor outcome of infants has been investigated through animal research, neurophysiological studies of neonates, and longitudinal follow-up of exposed infants. The inconsistency in reported findings may reflect methodological problems as well as variations among study populations and individual infants. Several studies using the Movement Assessment of Infants (MAI) have reported significant differences in motor performance at four months of age in infants who were cocaine-exposed prenatally, but specific clinical findings vary. A review of relevant work is presented here with a discussion of issues and variables which must be considered in an evaluation of the neuromotor consequences of intrauterine cocaine exposure for the developing infant. [Article copies available from The Haworth Document Delivery Service: 1-800-342-9678. E-mail address: getinfo@haworth.com]

INTRODUCTION

Since the increased use of cocaine by women of child-bearing age in the late 1980's, pediatric therapists have been involved with infants who

Marcia W. Swanson, MPH, PT, is affiliated with the Department of Rehabilitation Medicine, University of Washington Medical School, Seattle, WA 98195.

[Haworth co-indexing entry note]: "Neuromotor Outcome of Infants Exposed Prenatally to Cocaine: Issues of Assessment and Interpretation." Swanson, Marcia W. Co-published simultaneously in Physical & Occupational Therapy in Pediatrics (The Haworth Press, Inc.) Vol. 16, No. 1/2, 1996, pp. 35-50; and: Children with Prenatal Drug Exposure (ed: Lynette S. Chandler, and Shelly J. Lane) The Haworth Press, Inc., 1996, pp. 35-50. Single or multiple copies of this article are available from The Haworth Document Delivery Service [1-800-342-9678, 9:00 a.m. - 5:00 p.m. (EST). E-mail address: getinfo@haworth.com].

© 1996 by The Haworth Press, Inc. All rights reserved.

35

were exposed to cocaine in utero. Therapists who specialize in clinical evaluation of high-risk infants routinely assess infants who were prenatally exposed to cocaine and other illicit drugs. These infants comprise a substantial portion of follow-up clinic patients. In addition, infants with a history of prenatal cocaine exposure are frequently referred to therapists for developmental intervention, at times in the absence of abnormal clinical signs or symptoms.

Although presenting a challenging and intriguing new arena in which pediatric therapists can apply their clinical skills, the infant who was drug-exposed presents a dilemma for the conscientious therapist. Important questions, including accuracy of identification, potential labeling of children, and appropriate therapeutic management, are raised. Infants with documented, and, in some cases extensive, history of drug exposure throughout pregnancy often show no adverse effects and demonstrate normal development.[1-3] Other infants who exhibit abnormalities of reflexes, posture, and behavior within the first months of life demonstrate resolution of symptoms by six to twelve months of age without intervening.[4,5] Therapists can successfully adapt conventional pediatric therapeutic methods to treat the observed neuromotor abnormalities. A disturbing lack of knowledge exists, however, regarding the neurophysiologic basis for the tone and postural variations seen following cocaine exposure, their prognostic implications, and whether traditional therapeutic methods, such as those developed primarily for infants with cerebral palsy, are appropriate for this population.

To some extent, pediatric therapists may have inadvertently contributed to the popular view, described by medical personnel and educators and dramatized by the media, that infants exposed to cocaine prenatally are impaired and at risk for serious developmental consequences. As numerous investigators are now questioning early research and its conclusions,[6] therapists need to examine carefully the published literature regarding the effects of prenatal cocaine exposure on neuromotor outcome and to look critically and objectively at the infants with whom they work. This paper will review the relevant published information within the context of issues pertinent to therapists and their role with infants prenatally exposed to cocaine and other substances.

EFFECTS OF COCAINE ON NEUROMOTOR OUTCOME

Evidence for possible neuromotor consequences of prenatal cocaine exposure is available from at least three sources: animal studies, clinical or neurophysiologic research, and, to a lesser extent, longitudinal studies of infants.

Animal Studies

The findings of studies investigating the neurotoxic effects of prenatal cocaine exposure in rats and other animal models have been inconsistent. Although some researchers observed no effect of cocaine exposure on the maturation of righting reflexes,[7] others observed either delayed surface righting reflexes[8] or accelerated righting reactions[9] in rat pups who had been exposed to cocaine in utero. Cocaine exposure was associated with hyperactivity in some studies[8] while exposed pups in other investigations demonstrated hypoactivity.[10] A negative geotaxic test, which measures vestibular maturation and motor development, indicated marginal delay in one study of exposed pups;[11] no effect was observed in other investigations.[7,10] The variations in study results may be due to procedural differences including dosages, method of administration of cocaine, and timing of administration within the gestational and neonatal period. In general, locomotion and attainment of functional gross motor milestones have not shown significant effects as a result of cocaine exposure. Motor activity and exploratory behavior were not significantly altered in young or adult rats who were exposed to cocaine prenatally.[12] In a recent study,[13] however, cocaine was given to rodent pups during the neonatal period which is comparable to third-trimester exposure in humans. Exposed pups demonstrated impaired performance on tests of balance and coordination, as well as gait deviations.

Several important observations have been made by the investigators conducting animal studies. First, many of the neuromotor effects associated with cocaine exposure resolved as the exposed pups matured.[8,10] Second, in studies where abnormalities or deviations were found, they were not seen in all exposed animals but only in those who were given the highest dosages of drug.[10] Third, when differences were observed in cocaine-exposed pups, the findings could not be attributed with certainty to direct cocaine effects rather than to the consequences of toxicity and undernutrition in the mother.[10] Finally, there is the underlying question of the relevance of animal studies to human behavior and development. Although some researchers believe that there is "a close correspondence between humans and laboratory animals in the observed effects of known developmental toxicants,"[7,p.308] others state that "findings from animal studies generally relate poorly at best to human patterns of exposure."[14,p.297]

Clinical Studies

Human infants exposed to cocaine have been investigated for evidence of neurologic abnormalities. In one study, term infants prenatally exposed to cocaine and other drugs revealed a higher incidence of cranial abnormalities (intraventricular hemorrhage, echodensities, and cavitary lesions) than non-exposed high-risk or normal infants.[15] Although the lesions were located in areas of the brain that could influence motor function, including the basal ganglia, the infants demonstrated no clinical abnormalities in association with the lesions. In a subsequent study of very-low-birth-weight babies (<1500 grams), infants who were cocaine-exposed did not differ significantly from non-exposed infants in the incidence of Grades III and IV intraventricular hemorrhage or periventricular leukomalacia.[16] Recently, an association between prenatal cocaine exposure and bilateral caudate hemorrhage was found in the most heavily exposed neonates.[17]

EEG abnormalities were found in approximately one-half of a group of neonates exposed to cocaine prenatally;[4] however, this study did not include a control group and EEG findings were not associated with clinical abnormalities. Moreover, the EEG abnormalities normalized in all but one child during the first year of life. A similiar trend was observed in an investigation of brainstem transmission time in which infants who were cocaine-exposed demonstrated increased transmission time during the neonatal period but were similiar to matched controls by three to six months of age.[18] Although the incidence of EEG abnormalities in another cocaine-exposed sample was not significantly different from non-exposed infants, an analysis of behavioral state patterns in those who were drug-exposed revealed variations in sleep regulation, including precocious maturity of quiet sleep.[19] The implication of this observed sleep alteration is unclear.

Infant Studies

Early longitudinal investigations into the effects of in utero cocaine exposure reported alterations in reflex activity, motor control, and tremulousness during the neonatal period.[20,21] These studies, however, were often flawed by methodologic problems, including lack of a control group, unblinded examiners, and failure to control for confounding factors such as exposure to other substances in addition to cocaine. In recent neonatal studies in which experimental procedures have been more rigorous, cocaine effects on neurobehavioral measures, such as habituation and orientation, have not been consistently observed in the newborn period.[1-3,22-24] In two studies in which infants were followed beyond the first days of life, however, cocaine-exposed infants demonstrated neuromotor deviations in the areas of reflex activity and motor function at two to four weeks of age.[1,22] Kinematic analysis of the movements of cocaine-exposed subjects at one month of age revealed significant differences in head and arm, but not leg, movements.[25]

Most investigations of older infants who were prenatally exposed to cocaine have utilized the Bayley Scales of Infant Development (BSID) to evaluate outcome. They have generally reported no statistically significant differences in the BSID-Psychomotor Development Index (PDI) scores of cocaine-exposed infants, the majority of whom are functioning within the normal range at six, twelve and twenty-four months of age.[26-28] Similarly, a recent report stated that exposed and non-exposed groups were not significantly different in their performance on the Peabody Motor Quotient at 12 and 24 months.[29] At three years of age a group of children who were cocaine/polydrug-exposed were not significantly different from controls in mean scores on the Stanford-Binet scale but were significantly lower in their verbal reasoning.[30]

The strongest effects of prenatal cocaine exposure on motor outcomes were observed in a study of polydrug exposure using the Movement Assessment of Infants (MAI)[31] to assess neuromotor performance of infants at four months of age.[32] The risk for developmental delay was reported to be 40 times greater for those who were cocaine/polydrug-exposed than for non-exposed infants. Prenatal drug exposure was associated with increased risk of muscle tone abnormalities, persistence of primitive reflexes, and delayed volitional movement skills. Subsequent investigations using the MAI have not directly corroborated these early findings. In several studies in which cocaine-exposed infants have shown significant differences in MAI performance at four months of age,[33-35] the magnitude of variation is smaller and there are inconsistencies in the specific clinical findings. In one study,[33] infants who were cocaine-exposed differed in their average reflex and volitional movement scores, but muscle tone scores were not significantly different from controls. In contrast, another investigation reported that the only area of the MAI in which cocaine exposure produced significant differences was the automatic reactions subscale.[34] Finally, investigators in Boston reported no significant differences in MAI outcomes except in the volitional movement section, in which more heavily exposed infants had significantly *lower average risk scores* for volitional movement than unexposed or less heavily exposed infants.[35]

INTERPRETATION OF STUDY RESULTS

To establish a causal relationship between prenatal cocaine exposure and subsequent neuromotor deficits in infants, certain epidemiologic criteria must be met. These include: (1) biological plausibility; (2) strength of association; (3) dose-response relationship; and (4) consistency among various studies. The biologic pathways by which prenatal cocaine exposure could cause neurophysiologic damage have been extensively described.[36] Although a single mechanism has not been demonstrated, both the indirect effects of in utero cocaine exposure via vasoconstriction of maternal vascular supply and the direct neurotoxicity of cocaine in the fetal system could have an adverse impact on the developing fetal brain.

The remaining three criteria for a causal relationship have not been conclusively fulfilled by the studies conducted to date. Although the strong association between in utero cocaine exposure and abnormal neuromotor outcome reported by Schneider and Chasnoff[32] has not been replicated, three later studies found a statistically significant association between cocaine exposure and MAI performance at 4 months.[33-35] In at least two of these studies,[33,35] the significant association persisted after adjustment for various infant factors and other drugs used. The importance of controlling for potentially confounding factors in this population has been demonstrated in studies where an observed association has failed to reach statistical significance after adjustment for maternal and child variables.[1]

A linear dose-response relationship between the quantity of cocaine used and severity of motor impairment has not been reported for any longitudinal study evaluating infant outcome. Several studies have observed that sub-groups of infants who were exposed to greater quantities and/or duration of cocaine prenatally were more deviant from non-exposed infants than those who were less exposed.[33,35] Infants exposed through the third trimester of pregnancy had significantly higher average risk scores on the MAI than infants exposed only in the first one or two trimesters.[33] This supports earlier observations by Coles and colleagues[22] who found that duration of cocaine exposure was significantly related to neuromotor outcome at 28 days of age. The absence of a clear linear association may be related to the difficulty of accurately quantifying the amount of cocaine exposure during pregnancy because quantification of effective dose involves the quantity, frequency, and concentrations of active cocaine used by the mother as well as individual maternal and fetal metabolic factors.

Although the findings described provide support for a causal relationship between cocaine exposure and motor impairment, inconsistency among the results of various studies raises questions about the validity of the association observed. Longitudinal studies using the MAI have reported different patterns of neuromotor deviation with no two studies observing cocaine effects in the same sections of the MAI. Performance varied on individual items of the MAI as well. Schneider and Chasnoff[32] and Swanson[33] both reported that infants who were cocaine-exposed were significantly different from controls in the degree of tremulousness and tonic labyrinthine reflex in supine manifested. The two studies did not agree on other reflexes observed to be significantly different for cocaine-exposed and non-exposed groups. In the volitional movement section of the MAI, both studies observed less mature auditory and visual responses following cocaine-exposure. Schneider and Chasnoff[32] reported differences primarily in lower extremity activity, however, while Swanson[33] observed deviation in upper extremity function in infants who were co-caine-exposed.

Methodological Issues

Pediatric therapists who are working with infants who were drug-ex-posed must consider several important factors as they attempt to interpret the conclusions of these studies. The methodologic problems inherent in studies of the neurodevelopmental consequences of prenatal drug expo-sure have been discussed extensively.[6] Therapists reviewing the published reports of investigations of cocaine effects need to be knowledgeable about the basic criteria for valid research design and data analysis. Inade-quate sample size, non-masked examiners, or failure to provide a compari-son group that is similiar in its composition to the cocaine-exposed group can invalidate the conclusions of a study. When evaluating specific co-caine effects it appears to be particularly important to document and adjust for the presence of other drugs used by the mother during pregnancy. Jitteriness, a finding attributed to cocaine exposure in several preliminary studies, was found to be more highly associated with marijuana than with cocaine when the relative influence of these drugs was examined.[37] In other studies of infants exposed to multiple substances, alcohol was found to have the strongest effect on neonatal "withdrawal" signs and response to stress.[22,23] One researcher concluded, ". . . cocaine appeared to have a smaller impact on neonatal behavior than do alcohol, cigarettes, and/or marijuana."[22,p.29]

Even in recent longitudinal studies with well-designed protocols, the investigators acknowledge their inability to adequately control for poten-tial confounding factors such as prenatal care, maternal nutrition, and environmental influences on neurodevelopmental outcome. Moreover, ef-forts to compare the results of different studies are complicated by demo-graphic and geographical differences which include variations in drug composition, and patterns of drug use, including frequency, amount, and combinations of other drugs used concomitantly. For example, the subjects in the initial study using the MAI[32] were recruited from a drug-treatment program in Chicago which included predominantly heavy users of cocaine and other drugs. In contrast, the subjects in a later study conducted in Seattle[33] were recruited from a hospital-based maternity population which reflected a broad range of cocaine use from light to heavy. As a group, the infants in the Seattle study represented a less-heavily exposed cohort which may account for the fact that their total MAI risk scores were lower than those of the cocaine-exposed group in Chicago.

In addition to methodologic concerns that pertain to any longitudinal study of prenatal cocaine effects, there are issues specific to follow-up of neuromotor outcomes of which pediatric therapists must be particularly aware. These include instrumentation, variations in motor development based on race and culture, and asynchronous patterns of maturation.

Instruments for Assessment of Neuromotor Outcomes

Few instruments are available to assess subtle aspects of neuromotor development which may be affected by prenatal cocaine exposure. The BSID Psychomotor Scale is a relatively crude assessment of motor function which primarily evaluates the acquisition of motor milestones, not qualitative aspects of movement. The absence of significant findings in studies using the BSID as an outcome measure may be related to the limited and superficial scope of this tool.

The MAI[31] is the assessment tool which has been used most often to evaluate neuromotor outcomes of cocaine-exposure. The MAI provides a more comprehensive assessment of motor development because it includes items related to qualitative aspects of basic components of movement, muscle tone, primitive reflexes, and automatic reactions, as well as functional skills. The MAI has documented predictive validity with low birthweight infants for whom it is a more sensitive predictor of abnormal developmental outcome than the BSID Psychomotor Scale.[38,39] The capacity of the MAI to discriminate subtle differences in infant neuromotor behavior among diverse groups of infants has been demonstrated for infants with chronic lung disease, HIV infection, and other at-risk groups.[40-42] Consequently, the MAI is an appropriate and useful instrument for assessment of drug-exposure effects. Potential variation in the administration of the MAI may influence scores and therefore may contribute to observed discrepancies in study results.

Evaluation of the reliability of the MAI has indicated a range of reliabilities across sections and individual items.[43,44] In particular, the inter-rater reliability for the muscle tone section was determined to be "poor" in one analysis and was one of the least reliable sections in another analysis.

Muscle tone is the most subjective component of the MAI because it requires the examiner to manually palpate the extremities and observe the infant's spontaneous activity and then make a judgment regarding the quality of muscle tone. Given the subjectivity inherent in the muscle tone scores of different raters, the examiner's assumptions about the infant's overall risk status may influence the given score. Observer bias by examiners who were informed of infants' prenatal drug exposure status was demonstrated in a study involving examiner ratings of infants on videotape.[45] Such unintentional bias may have been a factor in the Chicago-based MAI study because examiners were not masked as to the infants' drug exposure history. The subjectivity of the examiners combined with low item reliability may have contributed to the significant difference between the muscle tone scores of exposed and non-exposed groups in this study which was not observed in other MAI studies.

A second aspect of the MAI involves the manner in which individual items are administered. The MAI is designed to be an extensive evaluation that enables the examiner to assess the infant's full capabilities. Sufficient time is provided to allow the infant repeated opportunities to perform a task. This presents two potential problems in the examination of the infant with drug exposure effects. First, the infant's successful performance of a task may depend on the skill and perseverance of the examiner. This may introduce variability in scores, particularly for high-risk infants for whom inter-rater reliability is less strong. As noted by Coles and associates,[22] an examiner's efforts towards achieving the infant's best response may work to obscure the negative effects of prenatal drug exposure on the infant's capabilities.

Secondly, the very length of the MAI evaluation, approximately 30 minutes, allows for more variation in the infant's response and, hence, more variability in scoring. Therapists report anecdotally that infants who were drug-exposed tend to be more unstable in their temperament and motor behavior. A typical description is one of a four-month-old infant who, when initially placed in backlying, lies with shoulders retracted, arms held back in an "airplane" posture, with hands open or fisted, while legs are extended in a low kick. Given this position, the examiner would give the child an abnormal muscle tone score on the MAI item, "Posture in Supine" because of the infant's apparent inability to move against gravity. It is not uncommon for the drug-exposed infant to show a very different response when again placed on his back later in the examination. At that time, he may round up his hips and shoulders, bringing his hands together in midline or to his knees without difficulty. Having observed this behavior, the examiner may now be inclined to rate the child's muscle tone in the supine position as "normal." The instructions in the MAI manual[31] do not specify how to score an infant who demonstrates such variability, which may be due to behavioral instability rather than true muscle tone fluctuation. This may reflect the instrument's original orientation towards the identification of infants with cerebral palsy, who tend to exhibit more static postures with less variation over time. In any case, the possibility for inconsistency among examiners, and hence among different longitudinal studies using the MAI as an outcome measure, remains an issue.

Racial and Cross-Cultural Variation

A second factor which requires attention when considering the motor outcome of cocaine-exposure is the racial composition of the sample. Neuromotor performance is distinct from cognitive function in that predetermined biologic differences between racial groups can impact the neurodevelopmental behavior of normally developing infants. Consequently, any investigation of cocaine effects must take these racial differences into account in both the study design and interpretation of results.

Numerous studies of cultural variations in motor development have concluded that black infants demonstrate increased muscle tone and advanced acquisition of gross motor skills, including standing.[46,47] In a cross-cultural study using the Neonatal Behavioral Assessment Scale (NBAS), Black infants demonstrated fewer startles and less tremulousness when compared to White infants.[48] The basis for the observed differences, whether they reflect variations in biologic endowment or in child-rearing practices, is debated. Whatever the reason, such racial differences could have an impact on the findings and conclusions of an investigation of cocaine effects. In one study using the BSID, non-white infants had significantly higher scores on the Psychomotor Scale than whites.[49] Furthermore, a cocaine effect, in which prenatal cocaine exposure was associated with *advanced* motor development, was observed in non-white infants but not in whites.[49] When the MAI is used as an outcome measure, studies which include predominantly Black infants, such as the Chicago[32] or Boston[35] studies, are likely to yield results of higher muscle tone, increased standing behavior (seen in the positive support reflex), and more advanced motor function than investigations of white infants. Moreover, to the extent that Black infants are over-represented in the cocaine-exposed group relative to the non-exposed group, an apparent cocaine effect of hypertonicity or advanced volitional movement could in fact result from the racial distribution between groups. To evaluate this potential source of bias on MAI scores, it is necessary to examine racial effects on item and section scores, as well as the total risk score, because the effect of increased muscle tone and persistent primitive reflexes on the total risk score could be obscured by precocious gross motor development.

In addition to specific effects of race, different child-rearing practices in given cultures have been associated with variations in motor development.[47,50] The impact of environmental influences is readily apparent to pediatric therapists who observe the effects of prolonged positioning in supine, use of a jumper or walker, or asymmetrical handling on the neuromotor development of an infant. Furthermore, specific maternal care practices associated with infant motor development have been found to be related to socioeconomic status.[51] Consequently, any differences observed in the neuromotor development of infants exposed to drugs must be considered within the context of the home environment, particularly if the mother is still involved with drugs. At the present time there is some evidence of the effect of environment on the cognitive development of infants whose mothers use cocaine. Path analysis of the Stanford-Binet performance of prenatally-exposed infants at three years of age revealed that home environment was as much of a contributing factor to IQ scores as prenatal drug exposure.[52] In another study,[53] infants living with their biologic mothers performed less well on language and play tasks than infants in foster care. At the present time, an environmental effect on the motor function of cocaine-exposed groups has not been described; however, a longitudinal study of infants exposed prenatally to methadone reported that delayed motor development at two years of age was associated with low familial socioeconomic status and lower maternal IQ scores.[54]

Patterns of Motor Development with Maturation

The results of both animal and infant studies of prenatal cocaine exposure suggest that neurologic and developmental abnormalities observed in the neonatal period tend to resolve as the infant matures making cocaine effects less evident with increasing age.[4,5,18] To the pediatric therapist this trend is similiar to the "transient dystonia" observed in low-birthweight infants. Up to 40% of all low-birthweight infants reportedly demonstrate neuromotor abnormalities of tone and reflexes in the first year of life, yet are considered to be neurodevelopmentally normal at one or two years of age.[55-57] This capacity for spontaneous resolution of observed abnormalities of tone and reflexes enables the pediatric therapist working with infants who were drug-exposed to maintain a positive and hopeful perspective regarding the child's potential outcome and to communicate a degree of optimism to the caregiver. At the same time, the therapist must recognize that any observed improvement in the infant's neurodevelopmental status may not be directly attributed to therapeutic intervention.

Long-term follow-up of low-birthweight infants with transient abnormalities reveals that, although neurologically normal at 12-24 months of age, they may be at increased risk for later neurodevelopmental disorders.[56-59] When compared to other children who were also low in birthweight but did not show abnormalities during the first year of life, children with a history of transient dystonia have been found to be at increased risk for school and learning problems, locomotor delay, and speech impairment.[56,58] Specific motor deficits that have been identified include those in fine motor function, visual-perceptual skills, and drawing tasks.[59] In a retrospective study comparing infants with moderately increased MAI risk scores at 4 months to a group of infants who had low-risk MAI scores at 4 months, outcome at 4 1/2 years differed only in significantly lower performance in pencil prehension for the infants with a history of higher risk.[60] At the present time, no longitudinal data exists on the predictive implications of tone and neuromotor abnormalities observed in cocaine-exposed groups. The findings with low-birthweight infants indicate the importance of on-going evaluation of fine motor, visual-motor and locomotor skills in these children as well as their behavior and learning.

CONCLUSION

Although there is legitimate concern about the impact of maternal cocaine use during pregnancy, the evidence supporting adverse effects of prenatal cocaine exposure on neuromotor outcome in infants is not conclusive when subjected to rigorous scientific review. Pediatric therapists must maintain an objective perspective relative to the debate on cocaine effects and with respect to the individual infants in their professional care who have a history of prenatal drug exposure. The longitudinal data currently available suggest the following: (1) Any negative consequences of prenatal cocaine exposure are likely to be subtle neuromotor deviations rather than gross developmental delay or abnormality. (2) Many or most exposed infants may be unaffected by in utero cocaine exposure; those who were most heavily exposed or exposed for the longest duration throughout pregnancy appear to be at highest risk for neuromotor impairment.[16,33,35] (3) The outcome for cocaine-exposure is highly individualized and reflects the synergistic interaction of many factors, including cumulative influence of the home environment on the older child. There is no typical or characteristic "cocaine-baby." (4) For infants who do show neuromotor deviations after prenatal exposure, current research reports do not reveal whether abnormalities will persist or if they are predictive of future neurodevelopmental problems.

The implications for the pediatric therapist are obvious. Decisions about intervention for an infant who was cocaine-exposed must be individualized and reflect realism about the degree of risk and the potential for positive outcome with or without therapy. In an era of diminishing resources, therapists need to ensure that their services are utilized only where clinically indicated and that necessary supportive services (education, social work, etc.), which may ultimately be more critical for the welfare of the child and family, are a priority. While communicating optimism about the potential for neurologically normal outcome, developmental monitoring into school age is required with particular attention to visual-motor, fine motor, and sensory orientation and processing. Finally, the pediatric therapist has the opportunity and the responsibility to promote and reinforce a positive and hopeful outlook on the part of caregivers and professionals and to discourage negative, biased, and uninformed predictions for the future of the developing child.

REFERENCES

1. Neuspiel DR, Hamel SC, Hochberg E, Greene J, Campbell D. Maternal cocaine use and infant behavior. *Neurotoxicology and Teratol.* 1991;13:229-233.
2. Richardson GA, Day NL. Maternal and neonatal effects of moderate cocaine use during pregnancy. *Neurotoxicology and Teratol.* 1991;13:455-460.
3. Woods NS, Eyler FD, Behnke M, Conlon M. Cocaine use during pregnancy: Maternal depressive symptoms and infant neurobehavior over the first month. *Inf Behav Dev.* 1993;16:83-98.
4. Doberczak TM, Shanzer S, Senie RT, Kandall SR. Neonatal neurologic and electroencephalographic effects of intrauterine cocaine exposure. *J Pediatr.* 1988;113:354-8.
5. Black M, Schuler M, Nair P. Prenatal drug exposure: Neurodevelopmental outcome and parenting environment. *J Ped Psych.* 1993;18:605-20.
6. Hutchings DE. The puzzle of cocaine's effects following maternal use during pregnancy: Are there reconcilable differences? *Neurotoxicol Teratol.* 1993;15:281-286.
7. Spear LP, Kirstein CL, Frambes NA. Cocaine effects on the developing central nervous system: Behavioral, psychopharmacological, and neurochemical studies. *Ann NY Acad Sci.* 1989;562:290-307.
8. Henderson MG, McMillen BA. Effects of prenatal exposure to cocaine or related drugs on rat developmental and neurological indices. *Brain Res Bull.* 1990;24:207-212.
9. Sobrian SK, Robinson NL, Burton LE, James H, Stokes DL, Turner LM. Neurobehavioral effects of prenatal exposure to cocaine. *Ann NY Acad Sci.* 1989;562: 383-386.

10. Church MW, Overbeck GW. Prenatal cocaine exposure in the Long-Evans rat: II. Dose-dependent effects on offspring behavior. *Neurotoxicol Teratol.* 1990; 12:335-343.

11. Kunko PM, Moyer D, Robinson SE. Intravenous gestational cocaine in rats: Effects on offspring development and weanling behavior. *Neurotoxicol Teratol.* 1993; 15:335-344.

12. Riley EP, Foss JA. Exploratory behavior and locomotor activity: A failure to find effects in animals prenatally exposed to cocaine. *Neurotoxicol Teratol.* 1991;13:553-558.

13. Barron S, Irvine J. Effects of neonatal cocaine exposure on two measures of balance and coordination. *Neurotoxicol Teratol.* 1994; 16:89-94.

14. Fantel AG. Puzzle of cocaine's effects following maternal use during pregnancy: Are there reconcilable differences? Commentary. *Neurotoxicol Teratol.* 1993;5:297.

15. Dixon SD, Bejar R. Echoencephalographic findings in neonates associated with maternal cocaine and methamphetamine use: Incidence and clinical correlates. *J Pediatr.* 1989;115:770-8.

16. Dusick AM, Covert RF, Schreiber MD et al. Risk of intracranial hemorrhage and other adverse outcomes after cocaine exposure in a cohort of 323 very low birth weight infants. *J Pediatr.* 1993;122:438-45.

17. Frank DA, McCarten K, Cabral H, Lenenson SM, Zuckerman BS. Association of heavy in utero cocaine exposure with caudate hemorrhage in term newborns. *Pediatr Res.* 1994;35:269A. Abstract.

18. Salamy A, Eldredge L, Anderson J, Bull D. Brain-stem transmission time in infants exposed to cocaine in utero. *J Pediatr.* 1990;117:627-629.

19. Legido A, Clancy RR, Spitzer AR, Finnegan LP. Electroencephalographic and behavioral-state studies in infants of cocaine-addicted mothers. *AJDC.* 1992;146:748-752.

20. Chasnoff IJ, Burns KA, Burns WJ. Cocaine use in pregnancy: Perinatal morbidity and mortality. *Neurotoxicol Teratol.* 1987;9:291-293.

21. Chasnoff IJ, Griffith DR, MacGregor S, Dirkes K, Burns KA. Temporal patterns of cocaine use in pregnancy: Perinatal outcome. *JAMA.* 1989;261:1741-1744.

22. Coles CD, Platzman KA, Smith I, James ME, Falek A. Effects of cocaine and alcohol use in pregnancy on neonatal growth and neurobehavioral status. *Neurotoxicol Teratol.* 1992;14:23-33.

23. Eisen LN, Field TM, Bandstra ES et al. Perinatal cocaine effects on neonatal stress behavior and performance on the Brazelton Scale. *Pediatrics.* 1991;88:477-480.

24. Mayes LC, Granger RH, Frank MA, Schottenfeld R, Bornstein MH. Neurobehavioral profiles of neonates exposed to cocaine prenatally. *Pediatrics.* 1993;91:778-783.

25. Fetters L, Tronick EZ. Kinematic analysis of the movements of in utero cocaine exposed one month old infants in different movement elicitation conditions. *Pediatr Res.* 1994;35:20A. Abstract.

26. Chasnoff IJ, Griffith DR, Freier C, Murray J. Cocaine/polydrug use in pregnancy: Two-year follow-up. *Pediatrics*. 1992;89:284-89.

27. Graham K, Feigenbaum A, Pastuszak A et al. Pregnancy outcome and infant development following gestational cocaine use by social cocaine users in Toronto, Canada. *Clin Invest Med*. 1992;15:384-394.

28. Van Baar AL, Fleury P, Ultee CA. Behaviour in first year after drug dependent pregnancy. *Arch Dis Child*. 1989;64:241-245.

29. Kilbride HW, Castor C, Rinck C. Two-year follow-up of term infants gestationally exposed to cocaine: Improved outcome with case management. *Pediatr Res*. 1994; 35:275A. Abstract.

30. Griffith DR, Azuma SD, Chasnoff IJ. Three-year outcome of children exposed prenatally to drugs. *J Am Acad Child Adolesc Psychiatry*. 1994;33:20-27.

31. Chandler LS, Andrews MS, Swanson MW. *Movement Assessment of Infants: A Manual*. Rolling Bay, WA: Authors; 1980.

32. Schneider JW, Chasnoff IJ. Motor assessment of cocaine/polydrug exposed infants at age 4 months. *Neurotoxicol Teratol*. 1992;14:97-101.

33. Swanson MW. *The Effects of Prenatal Cocaine Exposure on the Neuromotor Behavior of Infants at Four Months of Age*. Seattle, WA: University of Washington; 1992. Thesis.

34. Arendt R, Angelopoulos J, Bass O, Mascia J, Singer L. Sensory-motor development in four-month-old, cocaine exposed infants. *Pediatr Res*. 1994;35:18A. Abstract.

35. Rose-Jacobs R, Frank DA, Brown ER, Cabral H, Zuckerman BS. Use of the Movement Assessment of Infants (MAI) with in-utero cocaine-exposed infants. *Pediatr Res*. 1994;35:26A. Abstract.

36. Volpe JJ. Effect of cocaine use on the fetus. *New Eng J Med*. 1992; 327:399-407.

37. Parker S, Zuckerman B, Bauchner H, Frank D, Binci R, Cabral H. Jitteriness in full-term neonates: Prevalence and correlates. *Pediatrics*. 1990;85:17-23.

38. Harris SR. Early detection of cerebral palsy: Sensitivity and specificity of two motor assessment tools. *J Perinatol*. 1987;7:11-15.

39. Swanson MW, Bennett FC, Shy KK, Whitfield MF. Identification of neurodevelopmental abnormality at four and eight months by the Movement Assessment of Infants. *Dev Med Child Neurol*. 1992;34:321-337.

40. Swanson MW. Neuromotor assessment of low-birthweight infants with normal developmental outcome. *Dev Med Child Neurol*. 1989;31(suppl 59):27-28. Abstract.

41. Harris-Copp M. The HIV-infected child: A critical need for physical therapy. *Clin Management*. 1988;8:16-19.

42. Luther M, Ornstein M, Asztalos E. Predictive value of the Movement Assessment of Infants (MAI) and bronchopulmonary dysplasia as a confounding variable. *Pediatr Res*. 1992;31:254A. Abstract.

43. Harris SR, Haley SM, Tada WL, Swanson MW. Reliability of observational measures of the Movement Assessment of Infants. *Phys Ther*. 1984;64:471-475.

44. Brander R, Kramer J, Dancsak M, Marotta M, Stratford P, Chance G. Interrater and test-retest reliabilities of the Movement Assessment of Infants. *Pediatr Phys Ther.* 1993;5:9-15.

45. Eyler FD, Woods NS, Conlon M et al. Pygmalion in the cradle: Observer bias against cocaine-exposed infants. *Pediatr Res.* 1994;35:112A. Abstract.

46. Capute AJ, Shapiro BK, Palmer FB, Ross A, Wachtel RC. Normal gross motor development: The influences of race, sex, and socioeconomic status. *Dev Med Child Neurol.* 1985;27:635-643.

47. Cintas HM. Cross-cultural variation in infant motor development. *Phys Occ Ther Peds.* 1988;8(4):1-20.

48. Keefer CH, Tronick E, Dixon S, Brazelton TB. Specific differences in motor performance between Gusii and American newborns and a modification of the Neonatal Behavioral Assessment Scale. *Child Dev.* 1982;53:754-759.

49. Billman D, Nemeth P, Heimler R, Sasidharan P. Prenatal cocaine exposure (PCE): Effect of race on outcome. *Pediatr Res.* 1992;31:242A. Abstract.

50. Werner EE. Infants around the world: Cross-cultural studies of psychomotor development from birth to two years. *J Cross-Cultural Psychol.* 1972;3:11-134.

51. Plimpton CE, Regimbal C. Differences in motor proficiency according to gender and race. *Percept Motor Skills.* 1992;74:399-402.

52. Azuma SD, Chasnoff IJ. Outcome of children prenatally exposed to cocaine and other drugs: A path analysis of three-year data. *Pediatrics.* 1993;92:396-402.

53. Hurt H, Betancourt LM, Braitman LE, Malmud E, Brodsky NL, Giannetta JM. Progress report on the child with in utero cocaine (COC) exposure: Evaluations up to 30 months (m) of age. *Pediatr Res.* 1994;35:273A. Abstract.

54. Hans SL. Developmental consequences of prenatal exposure to methadone. *Ann NY Acad Sci.* 1989; 562:195-207.

55. Coolman RB, Bennett FC, Sells CJ, Swanson MW, Andrews MS, Robinson NR. Neuromotor development of graduates of the neonatal intensive care unit: Patterns encountered in the first two years of life. *Dev Behav Peds.* 1985;6:327-333.

56. Drillien CM, Thomson AJM, Burgoyne K. Low-birthweight children at early school-age: A longitudinal study. *Dev Med Child Neurol.* 1980;22:26-47.

57. Hack M, Caron B, Rivers A, Fanaroff AA. The very low birth weight infant: The broader spectrum of morbidity during infancy and early childhood. *Dev Behav Peds.* 1983;4:243-249.

58. Calame A, Reymond-Goni I, Maherzi M, Roulet M, Marchand C, Prodhomme LS. Psychological and neurodevelopmental outcome of high-risk newborn infants. *Helv Paed Acta.* 1976;31:287-297.

59. Ellison PH, Prasse DP, Siewart J, Browning CA. Correlations of neurologic assessment in infancy with fine motor, gross motor, and intellectual assessment at four years in a neonatal intensive care unit population. In: Stern L, Bard H, Friis-Hansen B, eds. *Intensive Care of the Newborn.* New York, NY: Masson;1983;4:241-246.

60. Stewart KB, Deitz JC, Crowe TK, Robinson N, Bennett FC. Transient neurologic signs in infancy and motor outcomes at 4 1/2 years in children born biologically at risk. *TECSE.* 1988;7:71-83.

Clinical Considerations in the Assessment of Infants and Young Children Affected by Parental Substance Abuse

Katherine B. Stewart
Pamela K. Richardson
Heather Carmichael Olson

SUMMARY. Focusing on families affected by parental substance abuse, this article discusses literature relevant to pediatric physical therapists and occupational therapists, describes examples of research assessment protocols, and offers a number of clinical considerations for in-depth assessment of this population. Based on what we currently know as a result of empirical studies, and what we have learned clinically from infants and families affected by substance abuse, recommendations are made for pediatric physical therapy and occupational therapy assessments of this infant population. Pediatric

Katherine B. Stewart, MS, OTR, is Clinical Associate Professor, School of Occupational Therapy, University of Puget Sound, Tacoma, WA 98416. Pamela K. Richardson, MS, OTR, is Research Examiner, MOM's Project, and doctoral student, College of Education, University of Washington, Seattle, WA 98416. Heather Carmichael Olson, PhD, is Research Assistant Professor, Department of Psychiatry and Behavioral Sciences, School of Medicine, University of Washington, Seattle, WA 98195.

The authors wish to acknowledge the families participating in the MOM's Project for their contributions and willingness to share their perspectives.

This work was partially supported by a grant from the National Institute of Drug Abuse, #06361-05.

[Haworth co-indexing entry note]: "Clinical Considerations in the Assessment of Infants and Young Children Affected by Parental Substance Abuse." Stewart, Katherine B., Pamela K. Richardson, and Heather Carmichael Olson. Co-published simultaneously in *Physical & Occupational Therapy in Pediatrics* (The Haworth Press, Inc.) Vol. 16, No. 1/2, 1996, pp. 51-72; and: *Children with Prenatal Drug Exposure* (ed: Lynette S. Chandler, and Shelly J. Lane) The Haworth Press, Inc., 1996, pp. 51-72. Single or multiple copies of this article are available from The Haworth Document Delivery Service [1-800-342-9678, 9:00 a.m. - 5:00 p.m. (EST). E-mail address: getinfo@haworth.com].

© 1996 by The Haworth Press, Inc. All rights reserved.

51

therapists may wish to consider a transactional developmental model that includes examination over time of the biologic, environmental, and interactional risk and protective factors in infants and young children. *[Article copies available from The Haworth Document Delivery Service: 1-800-342-9678. E-mail address: getinfo@haworth.com]*

With the increasing number of early identification programs and the rising incidence of drug abuse during pregnancy,[1,2] physical therapists and occupational therapists are assessing a growing population of infants and young children who are developmentally at-risk because of parental substance abuse. As pediatric therapists evaluate more infants and children affected by parental substance abuse, clinical questions arise regarding the appropriateness of traditional motor assessments and the need for modifications. The purpose of this article is three-fold: to summarize relevant information from the literature about the prenatal risks and postnatal experiences of infants and children in substance-using families; to discuss how infant and caregiver assessment protocols are being carried out in a Seattle-based research project; and to present clinical considerations pertinent to physical therapy and occupational therapy assessments of infants affected by parental substance abuse.

DEVELOPMENTAL OUTCOME AND RISK FACTORS

Data describing infant outcome and the quality of caregiving among families in which there is prenatal substance abuse suggest the need for careful, comprehensive, longitudinal assessment of this very diverse at-risk population.[3,4] Prenatal alcohol or illicit drug exposure can have pervasive effects on child and family outcome. Not only are there possible direct effects on the child, but, especially if substance abuse continues after the child's birth, there can potentially be effects on child-caregiver interactions and the environment in which the child is raised. Given the complexity of this clinical problem, Zuckerman and Bresnahan[5] suggest that children prenatally exposed to and possibly affected by alcohol or other drugs are "doubly vulnerable." They propose that a transactional model of development be used to understand developmental outcomes in this population. The transactional model, originally described by Sameroff and Chandler,[6] suggests that developmental outcome results from the ongoing and dynamic interaction between an individual child and his or her experiences in the social and physical environment. Consistent with the transactional model, Greenspan and Meisels[7] articulate what they term a "new vision" for the assessment of infants and young children that includes an integrated developmental approach. When applying the transactional developmental approach to assessments of infants prenatally exposed to alcohol or other drugs, therapists not only carefully evaluate the infant's neurodevelopmental and neurobehavioral status, but also consider the infant's social and physical experiences and how the infant's characteristics in turn shape those experiences over time. To provide a comprehensive understanding of the infant's development, pediatric therapists should go beyond the assessment of the infant's neurodevelopmental status and consider what Belsky[8] describes as the "goodness of fit" between the infant and his or her environment.

As stated by Griffith and Freier,[9(p.229)] "many drug-using women share several characteristics that researchers have found to interfere with parenting abilities of drug-free women and may affect the long-term outcome of their children." These characteristics include a high percentage of chemically-dependent women who can be classified as having low socioeconomic status, living in high-stress environments, and experiencing psychopathology. Other authors including Reed,[10] Davis,[11] and Zaichkin and Houston[12] have commented on the relatively frequent occurrence of maternal depression, history of childhood trauma, lack of positive parental role models, ambivalence toward childrearing, and lack of parenting and social support among women using drugs during pregnancy.

Although the vulnerability of this population as a whole has been documented, it is critical to note that not all children who experience prenatal exposure to substance abuse show physical, developmental, or social-emotional difficulties as a result. A great deal of variability exists in the type and severity of illicit drug and alcohol effects in children, and there are clear individual differences in how infants and children respond to family environments affected by substance use. In fact, families themselves respond in different ways to substance use and to the recovery process. Myers and colleagues[13] support a risk model rather than a deficit model for use in understanding developmental outcomes in this population. Biologic, environmental, and interpersonal risk factors must be considered along with the equally important protective factors in these infants and families. The important point is that the strengths of the infant, caregiver, and environment must be considered along with the deficits in order to obtain a complete assessment.

A Brief Review of Biological Risk Factors

Most substance abusers are involved in polydrug use. Illicit drug use is typically paired with cigarette smoking and drinking alcohol. Even used alone, the "legal drugs" of nicotine and alcohol can have adverse effects on the developing fetus. It is clearly established that gestational tobacco use is related to lowered birth weight, a biological risk factor, although the impact of tobacco on early learning and long-term functional effects are less clear.[14] Alcohol is a common and well-recognized neurobehavioral teratogen which can have long-term consequences for development of an affected individual. The most serious impact of heavy alcohol use during pregnancy is seen in Fetal Alcohol Syndrome (FAS), a developmental disability that is currently estimated to occur in 1.9 per 1000 live births.[15] Defining characteristics of FAS include pre- or postnatal growth retardation, characteristic craniofacial abnormalities, and variable evidence of central nervous system (CNS) dysfunction.[16] In infants, the CNS involvement is variable and may include irritability, hypotonia, difficulty with sucking, and in some cases, failure to thrive.[17,18] In a review of the FAS literature with implications for physical therapists, Osborn and colleagues[19] reported evidence of neurodevelopmental abnormalities in infants and children with FAS, including alterations in reflex behavior, less mature motor behavior, and decreased ability to habituate. The early signs of FAS are the first indication of a documented, lifelong pattern of developmental and/or functional deficits with widely varying levels of individual ability.

Kaltenbach and Finnegan[20] report a high incidence of neonatal abstinence syndrome in infants born to mothers who are opiate-dependent. This syndrome is a generalized disorder characterized by hyperirritability, gastrointestinal dysfunction, respiratory distress, and vague autonomic symptoms that include yawning, sneezing, mottling, and low-grade fever. The infant may also exhibit feeding difficulties, tremors, high-pitched crying, and increased muscle tone. Although there may be continuing neurobehavioral impairment over the early days of life, the long-term outcome of prenatal exposure to opiates remains in question. Wilson[21] concludes that heroin use during pregnancy is not associated with major developmental disability or a specific behavioral syndrome, and that other biological and environmental factors (especially those inherent in the lifestyle of a drug-dependent parent) have an important impact on the behavior and cognitive performance of heroin-exposed children.

Daltiero and Fried,[22] acknowledging the need for more data, describe subtle neonatal effects of marijuana exposure, such as increased tremors, frequently accompanied by exaggerated startles, and some increased irritability and impaired visual habituation. They also discuss a subtle, possible delaying, effect of prenatal marijuana exposure on at least some aspects of nervous system maturation. Clear, negative effects of prenatal marijuana exposure were not seen at 12 and 24 months of age. Consequently, the impact of marijuana exposure in utero may be transitory, or the cognitive effects may manifest later in life when more complex demands are placed on nervous system functions. Interactive effects of lifestyle risk factors are important in understanding the impact of gestational marijuana use on child outcome.

Findings on early cocaine effects are not always consistent, nor free of methodological limitations; initial speculations of drastic effects have not, however, been confirmed.[23] Cocaine-related problems may include preterm birth, transient neurophysiologic abnormalities such as hypertonicity and tremulousness, poor feeding, and neurobehavioral difficulties such as impairment in the affected infant's interactive and organizational abilities.[5,11,19,24,25] The long-term significance of these early problems is still under study.[26] Zuckerman and Frank[27] suggest that prenatal exposure to cocaine is a potential but not inevitable developmental insult.

Although it is commonly believed that prenatal exposure to drugs results in negative developmental outcomes, Coles and Platzman[28] report a review of data from various investigations that suggest a wide range of effects in infants exposed in utero to teratogenic or toxic substances. Clearly much more research must be done to understand the developmental outcome of exposure to illicit drugs before birth. The picture cannot be oversimplified; prenatal exposure to drugs, genetic contributions, and environmental factors together shape the child's developmental outcome.[29]

Environmental Risk Factors

Environmental risk factors in children exposed before birth to alcohol or illicit drugs are not usually a primary reason for referral to physical therapists or occupational therapists. Pediatric therapists, however, must be acutely aware of the role these environmental risk factors play in the dynamics of child development. Some of the factors that can put infants at environmental risk include continued maternal substance abuse or the struggle of recovery, parental psychopathology, and poverty.

Few studies have specifically investigated the impact of parenting behavior of substance abusers on young children's development. Some investigators suggest that if the primary caregiver of the infant continues to abuse alcohol or other drugs the likelihood of suboptimal caregiving within a chaotic environment increases.[8,30]

Kaplan-Sanoff and colleagues[31] discuss the relationship between poverty and child outcomes by examining the effects of extremely stressful environments such as maternal drug use on child development. A drug-seeking environment can often be characterized by financial problems, trouble with violence or legal involvement, multiple moves, medical problems, and generally high stress levels. Even the environment of a woman in recovery from chemical dependence can be stressful though hopeful, as she struggles with drug cravings, changes in her social support network and daily activities, and alterations in perceptions of her children and herself.

Women who abuse substances tend to exhibit guilt, shame, anxiety, depression, and low self-esteem, and may show co-occurring psychiatric conditions.[10,11,29] Increasing amounts of evidence suggest that maternal mental health disorders place infants and young children at increased risk for developmental problems. For example, some studies suggest that patterns of parent-child interaction differ among depressed mothers, depending on chronicity, severity, or other risk factors, but the interaction patterns observed could impede an infant's sense of control, pleasure, and feelings of security with the mother.[32] Maternal depression serves to limit the physical and emotional energy affected mothers can invest in parenting.[33]

Poverty is another environmental risk factor common in many families affected by substance abuse. Kaplan-Sanoff and colleagues[31] state that the biologic risks of poverty, such as malnutrition, limited access to health care, and increased childhood illnesses, and psychosocial risks, such as inadequate social supports, single parenting, and parental unemployment, each serve to place children at additional risk for adverse developmental outcomes.

Risk Factors in Caregiver-Infant Interactions

Important links have been discovered between certain aspects of caregiver-infant interactions and the infant's development.[34] Researchers and clinicians have expressed concern that ongoing maternal substance abuse may pose a hazard to infant-caregiver interactions, and that a child experiencing fetal alcohol or drug effects may be difficult to parent.[35] A small number of studies with chemically-dependent women have found that they often display a sense of lessened parental competence and/or gaps in childrearing knowledge, but have similarities with normative data or a comparison group on many other parenting attitudes.[29] Families affected by substance abuse appear to experience more risk factors which are associated with child maltreatment,[36] but the cause-effect relationship (and intervening factors) between substance use and child maltreatment is only now under study.[36-39] Some evidence, often among women dependent on opiates and their children, but also among women using cocaine, suggests the presence of interactive impairments and/or decreased mutual enjoyment within the dyad.[40,41] Evidence among polydrug users also suggests that no caregiver-child interaction differences occur when comparisons are made to non-using dyads.[42] This issue definitely needs further study. It is possible that dyadic coordination or "goodness-of-fit" between parent and child may be a problem in at least some families affected by substance abuse, especially given the reported higher incidence of maternal depression which can affect infant-caregiver interaction.

Clearly individual diversity exists in this population, and an assumption that substance use inevitably leads to poor parenting should be avoided. As Mayes[29] recommends, research is still needed to document whether some substance-abusing parents do in fact have impaired relationships with their children and, if so, how these patterns of relatedness differ from those in other families not affected by substance abuse, but who are disadvantaged or living in stressful environments.

It is important to emphasize again that while prenatal alcohol or illicit drug exposure puts infants and young children in "double jeopardy," many children in this at-risk population do not exhibit symptoms of drug or alcohol effects. A "rush to judgment" with an assumption that all drug-exposed children will do poorly is not appropriate.[25] Toxins and teratogens, such as cocaine and alcohol, do not affect all exposed offspring, and there are clear individual differences and variability in the effects that do occur. The environment has variable effects on child development as well. In addition, some children from disorganized and highly stressful environments appear to be resilient to the development of psychopathology. Investigators such as Werner[43] and Luthar and Zigler[44] have examined why resilient children do well in spite of poor conditions, and they suggest identifying possible protective factors within the environment that can be put in place to assist those children who are more vulnerable.

Pediatric physical therapists and occupational therapists, along with other health professionals, should bear in mind the transactional model of development and look for and build upon the strengths in infants and families affected by substance abuse. Professionals working with this population must learn to assess both the risk factors and the protective factors within the child, as well as the child's environment, to gain a full picture of the child's strengths and areas of concern.

ASSESSMENT PROTOCOLS FOR THE MOM's PROJECT

Pediatric therapists working with the population of drug-exposed children currently face two formidable tasks: (1) developing assessment protocols that yield accurate and useful data; and (2) implementing these protocols in an effective and sensitive manner. The application of a transactional model of development to a set of assessment protocols currently being implemented in the MOM's Project is described below as one example of how therapists can begin to meet these challenges.

The MOM's Project is a Seattle-based intervention and research project funded by the National Institute on Drug Abuse, with additional support from the Washington State Division of Alcohol and Substance Abuse, and participation of Washington State's Department of Social and Health Services, the King County Division of Alcohol and Substance Abuse, and several non-profit parenting agencies. Part of a nationwide research effort, the MOM's Project was designed to investigate the effects of comprehensive services, including gender-appropriate alcohol/drug treatment, as well as medical, case management, and family support services, on outcomes among chemically-dependent pregnant women and their children. Among the questions explored were the characteristics of women entering treatment, who stays in or drops out of treatment, whether treatment is helpful for participating families, and the characteristics of families who do poorly and well after intervention. An equally important contribution of the MOM's Project lies in a description of the innovative services offered to participating women and children, and in the clinical wisdom gathered in the effort to provide appropriate assessment and treatment of this at-risk and understudied population.

Participants in the MOM's Project were pregnant women aged 16 years or older who were at less than 28 weeks gestation when entering the study and had a demonstrated chemical dependency problem. MOM's Project participants agreed to participate in follow-up developmental research visits, and in other types of data collection. The first-year follow-up visits occurred in a university child development clinic setting scheduled when the infants were around four months and twelve months of age, corrected for prematurity, with some variation in the actual age at which individual children were seen. With no access to earlier records or to treatment personnel, the examiners in this study were "blind" to the caregiver's gestational exposure history, treatment status, information about current drug/alcohol use, and the results of any prior developmental testing of the infant or psychosocial assessment of the mother. In addition, the interrater reliability of all measures was checked on a periodic basis.

Data collection for the follow-up phase of the project is ongoing. To date, a total of 96 cases have been seen at the four-month infant visit, and 55 cases have been seen at both the four-month and twelve-month infant visits. To better understand the rationale for the development and implementation of the assessment protocols, demographics of the 96 cases seen at the four-month infant visit are briefly described. These are preliminary data and do not represent the total expected sample for the MOM's Project. At time of enrollment into the study, the average age of these 96 mothers was 26.5 years and ranged from 16 years to 41 years, with about 14% less than 21 years old. Over one-third of these 96 cases (which included teenagers still in school) had not completed high school at study entry. About one-third of these 96 women had graduated from high school or received a G.E.D. and one-fourth had some post-secondary education. The women's average reading level was at the sixth grade level, with much variability. About 46% of these 96 women reported their ethnicity as Caucasian, 43% as African-American, 4% as Native American, and the remainder considered themselves biracial or of other ancestry. Based on self-report when entering the study, over half had never been married, about 28% were separated, widowed, or divorced, and about 11% were either married or living with a partner. While pregnant with the target child at study entry, 26% had no other living children, 54% had one or two living children, and the remainder had three or more offspring. These older children were not necessarily in their birth mother's custody. Most of the women were polydrug users, with their individual primary drug of choice ranging across alcohol, cocaine/crack, heroin, marijuana, and other illicit drugs. Of the 96 caregivers bringing infants to the 4-month visit, 80% were birth mothers, 9% were caregivers from the infants' extended families, 9% were foster parents, one was a pre-adoptive mother, and one was a birth father. Of the 55 caregivers bringing infants to the 12-month visit, 69% were birth mothers, 15% were caregivers from the infants' extended families, 13% were foster parents, three were adoptive mothers, and two were biological fathers. Test results and information on infant characteristics are not yet available.

Measures Used for the MOM's Project Follow-Up Visits

Based on prior studies of children prenatally exposed to alcohol or illicit drugs, our clinical experience, and specific research questions under investigation in the MOM's Project, the third author, a study investigator, developed in-depth assessment protocols for each of the caregiver-infant visits. Given the biological and environmental vulnerability of the infants in this study, thorough assessment protocols were devised and are fully described in the following sections as examples for therapists interested in assessing this population of at-risk children. To assess these infants within a transactional developmental frame of reference, a combination of clinical and standardized measures were selected. Contextual measures including maternal psychosocial status (e.g., maternal depression, coping, social support, and life stress) affecting the child and the quality of the caregiving environment at home were assessed in other phases of the MOM's Project. *Four-Month Follow-Up Protocol.* The four-month infant follow-up visits were conducted by the first author. The length of the visit was approximately two to two-and-one-half hours depending on the infant's and caregiver's pace in completing the measures. To assess the infants' developmental status, the Bayley Scales of Infant Development (BSID), including the Mental Scale, Motor Scale and Infant Behavior Record (IBR),[45] were administered first. The IBR is a descriptive rating scale that provides information about the infant's behavior patterns, including interpersonal and affective domains, as well as qualitative observations of behavior. The BSID was followed immediately by the Movement Assessment of Infants Screening Tool (MAIST)[46] which briefly assesses the neurodevelopmental status of the infant. The MAIST is used to screen infants from 2 months to 12 months of age for comparison with normative data for those ages.

The caregiver was next provided with a standardized set of toys and asked to play with the infant as she normally does at home. This unstructured play sequence was eight minutes in length and was videotaped by a research assistant with a camera in the room to obtain adequate views of the parent and child's affective interchange. Next, the Nursing Child Assessment Satellite Training (NCAST) Teaching Scale[47] was administered. The NCAST Teaching Scale rates the responsiveness of the child and caregiver to each other during a structured teaching interaction usually lasting from one to six minutes. Caregivers are rated on sensitivity to cues, alleviating distress, and cognitive and social-emotional growth fostering. Children are rated on the ability to produce clear cues and the amount of responsiveness to the caregiver. After administration of the NCAST Teaching Scale, the caregiver was asked to tend to the infant as necessary while the examiner scored the "in vivo" NCAST data. These naturalistic caregiving events, which were videotaped from behind an observation mirror, often consisted of feeding, comforting, or changing the infant. To obtain a more comprehensive neuromotor assessment, those items on the Movement Assessment of Infants (MAI)[48] not on the MAIST were also administered.

The rest of the research visit included an interview with the caregiver regarding the infant's home environment and developmental concerns, and the infant's health. Questions addressed daily caregiving routines, including who provided caregiving on a regular basis; regulation of feeding and sleeping schedules; discussion of concerns in the areas of vision, hearing, physical, mental, and social development; and medical history, including continuity of medical care, immunizations, illnesses, and accidents that could potentially affect development. Caregivers were also asked to describe their child's personality, what they enjoyed about their child, and their hopes for their child in the future. Toward the end of the visit, the Parenting Stress Index-Short Form (PSI-SF)[49] was administered. This brief, written questionnaire explores caregiver stress in relation to parenting, the child, and the parent-child interaction. The child's weight, length, and head circumference were measured and entered on a growth chart to obtain age percentile scores. Immediately following the visit, the examiner rated such constructs as the quality of infant development and mother-infant interaction, and the frequency of unusual behaviors potentially evident among infants affected by drugs, such as rigid muscle tone when environmental stimulation is high, excessive crying, visual over-fixation on objects in the environment, and spontaneous startles.

Two areas of clinical consideration are highlighted here as especially important in work with families affected by parental substance abuse. First, infants and their caregivers perform more optimally when the examiner addresses the emotional and physical needs of both the infant and the caregiver throughout the examination. Second, when caregivers are offered respect and brief but relevant information about their infants throughout the exam, they are more engaged in the assessment and better able to recognize the individual strengths and needs of their infants.

In the MOM's Project, care was taken to set up the testing environment and administer the measures in a manner responsive to the physical and emotional needs of both caregiver and the infant. For the physical comfort of the caregivers, nutritious snacks were available throughout the visit and a couch was placed conveniently in the testing room. To ease feelings of anxiety common to all parents who undergo testing of their infant, the examiner first briefly introduced herself and her testing qualifications, and then fully explained the purpose of the visit. The caregiver was encouraged to ask questions at any time and take a break from the interaction, if needed. The person videotaping the sessions was introduced at the session's start so the caregiver knew exactly who would be observing the examination. During testing, the examiner paid close attention to the pace of the exam, making sure the infant was physically handled and positioned in a manner that promoted optimal performance. When the infant became fussy and could not be consoled through close physical comfort, then the caregiver either fed or allowed the infant to nap. Throughout the visit the caregivers were provided with specific information about the infant's relative strengths and needs. For example, during the test item of posture in prone on the Movement Assessment of Infants, the examiner might say, "Wow! Look how you can keep your head up so you can look at Mom!," or, when the infant started to fuss, the examiner might say, "It looks like you're having a hard time paying attention. Would it help if I turned the lights down?"

Twelve-Month Follow-Up Protocol. The 12-month infant visits were carried out by the second author and were also two to two-and-one-half hours long. The BSID was administered to assess developmental status, consistent with the four-month examination. The caregiver was then given a standardized and age-appropriate toy set, and again asked to play with the child as she typically does at home. Videotaping of this eight-minute unstructured play sequence took place from an observation room with a one-way mirror, and these videotaped data are being coded in several ways. (One tool that is clinically useful for coding videotaped interactions is the Parent/Caregiver Involvement Scale.[50] The P/CIS provides a global assessment of the amount, quality and appropriateness of the caregiver's involvement with the child with a focus on interactive patterns of the caregiver which are likely to foster optimal development in the child.)

The NCAST Teaching Scale was administered next, and, while the examiner scored the NCAST data, the caregiver was asked to tend to the infant as needed. These naturalistic caregiving events were also video-taped from behind an observation mirror. Three questionnaires that focus on perceptions of parenting were then administered. The PSI-SF tapped parenting attitudes, as in the four-month infant follow-up visit. Other questionnaires tapped information relevant to parenting effectiveness and included the Child Abuse Potential Inventory (CAPI)[51] which assess parental risk for child maltreatment, and the Adult-Adolescent Parenting Inventory (AAPI)[52] which taps constructs such as inappropriate developmental expectations and parent-child role reversal. The remainder of the research visit included interviews on health, developmental concerns, and the child's home environment. Caregivers were also asked to rate the helpfulness of a number of supports and resources as protective factors in raising their child. If there were biological siblings and the caregiver knew them well, she was asked to rate how the siblings were doing. Caregivers were also given the opportunity to talk about their child's personality, what they enjoyed about their child, and their hopes for the child's future. Child growth was measured and recorded on a growth chart.

The Early Coping Inventory (ECI)[53] was completed following the 12-month infant visit, based on the examiner's observations of the child's behavior during the varied situations of the visit. The ECI measures the ability of children aged 4 to 36 months to cope with everyday environmental stresses. Coping behaviors are rated in three areas: sensory-motor, reactive behavior, and self-initiated behavior. The ECI examines both strengths and weakness in children's coping abilities, and information from the ECI can be used in intervention planning. Consistent with the four-month visit protocol, the examiner at the 12-month visit rated the constructs of the quality of infant development and the caregiver-infant interaction, and the frequency of unusual behaviors potentially evident among infants with drug effects.

During the 12-month infant visits, as in earlier visits, meeting the physical and emotional needs of the caregivers and infants, and offering information and asking questions in a non-judgmental, respectful way, seemed crucial in working effectively with families affected by parental substance abuse. Test items that required the active involvement of the child were completed early in evaluation, while the child's attention and motivation were at an optimal level. When necessary, the order of the testing protocol was adjusted to meet the needs of the child and/or caregiver. During the approximately 20 minutes it took the caregivers to fill out the questionnaires, the examiner watched or played with the child, eliciting information for the ECI and allowing the caregiver to work without interruption. During this informal play and observation time, the examiner could assess the child's preferred play activities, attention span, communication, motor and social skills, coping behaviors, and frustration tolerance in an unstructured situation.

Examiners were sensitive to the caregivers' needs regarding the completion of written questionnaires. In a respectful way, caregivers were offered assistance in completing the questionnaires if they appeared to be having difficulty in reading, or if the need to physically comfort a fussy infant affected their ability to complete the questionnaires.

The testing situation was also seen as an opportunity for caregiver and examiner to learn from one another about the infant's capabilities. Caregivers were asked whether they viewed their child's performance as typical, and what skills were not demonstrated during testing. The examiner described emerging or unexpected abilities demonstrated by the child, and provided anticipatory guidance to the caregiver about skills upcoming for the child. Testing also became a time when play materials were discussed. Caregivers often questioned the examiner about what toys were appropriate for their child and where to purchase them. The examiner was able to provide advice on age-appropriate toys and about purchasing or making toys that would serve a variety of play purposes, as well as, interest and challenge the child over a long period of time.

At the end of the 12-month session, the caregiver was given a feedback form which summarized clearly and briefly findings about the child, along with the child's measurements and brief, practical suggestions on how to facilitate further development. Although intervention was not a goal of these research visits, both the examiners' and caregivers' concerns and questions were addressed honestly and in a straightforward manner as they arose. The examiner discussed the significance of important or troubling child behaviors and briefly suggested ways to handle them. Realistic developmental expectations of the child were discussed. Caregivers were reinforced for positive parenting skills demonstrated during the session, with comments such as, "That was so nice the way you answered her back when she babbled to you. That's how she'll learn about having a conversation with another person," or, "You really are aware of some nice ways to comfort him when he gets upset. He responds really well when you hold him that way." This was done to assist caregivers in becoming more aware of actions helpful with children who could be challenging to parent and to highlight the effects of caregivers' behaviors and interactions with their children.

CLINICAL CONSIDERATIONS FOR PEDIATRIC THERAPISTS

The process of administering the four-month and twelve-month infant assessments for the MOM's Project provided the research examiners an important opportunity to learn about infants prenatally exposed to alcohol or drugs and their caregivers. The following section discusses clinical considerations that grew out of the authors' assessment experience and could be valuable to other pediatric therapists working with this population.

The expertise of pediatric physical therapists and occupational therapists may best be used in comprehensive assessments of infants and young children first identified as delayed on basic developmental screening conducted by primary health care providers or early childhood personnel. Similar to Lane's[54] recommendations, our clinical experience on the MOM's Project suggests that pediatric therapy assessment should include developmental and behavioral measures of the infant, evaluation of the infant's coping skills through tools such as the ECI, assessment of the caregiver-infant interactions during functional tasks such as feeding, dressing, and playing, and an interview with the caregiver regarding concerns, perceptions of parenting and the infant's development and behavior, and other contextual issues. Pediatric therapists working with this population should consider expanding their repertoire of assessment tools to include the evaluation of the infant's social environment (e.g., quality of caregiver-infant interactions, caregiver perceptions of infant's abilities, availability of a strong attachment figure, supports available to the family).

Depending on the assessment purposes, setting, and therapist skills, the assessment protocol will vary. The assessment protocols used for the MOM's Project were designed for research visits, each 2 1/2 hours in length. Assessment methods and measures used in clinics and early intervention programs may differ as a result of time constraints and other factors. Nevertheless, for any assessment of this complex population, a carefully selected combination of standardized tools, clinical observations, and caregiver interview is strongly recommended.[7,8]

The design of the comprehensive assessment protocols for the MOM's Project was based on the transactional model of child development. As in the assessment of children with other pediatric diagnoses (e.g., prematurity, Down syndrome, spina bifida, cerebral palsy), therapists should carefully consider the emerging skills at each phase of the infant's development and use multiple measures when assessing infants and children with prenatal alcohol or drug exposure. For example, at the four-month infant visit for the MOM's Project, infant neuromotor abilities were examined in depth via the BSID* and the MAI. At the 12-month infant visit, infant behavior was scrutinized using the IBR, the ECI, and specially-designed clinical rating scales. Pediatric therapists who follow children into their toddler and preschool years should consider careful analysis of sensorimotor integration, play and feeding behaviors, and the ability to self-regulate. Pediatric therapy assessment tools useful for this older age group may include the Miller Assessment for Preschoolers,[55] the Transdisciplinary Play-Based Assessment,[56] and the Observational Scale for Mother-Infant Interaction During Feeding.[57] Child behavior problems and the "goodness-of-fit" between caregiver and child should also be considered. In consultation with a psychologist or educator, the pediatric therapist may wish to use the Child Behavior Checklist for Ages 2-3.[58]

Because parents with a history of substance abuse come from a variety of socioeconomic and ethnic backgrounds, therapists must be culturally competent and careful to avoid inappropriate value judgments about parental skills and knowledge. When providing information about the child, a skillful therapist carefully adapts both verbal and nonverbal communication to meet the needs and style of the caregivers. Given the multicultural and diverse demographic makeup of participants in the MOM's project, the examiners found it most effective to take a broad range of cultural and individual differences into consideration, and to adopt a flexible, open, and accepting but realistic attitude.

When assessing this population, the importance of an interdisciplinary

---

*The reader should note that a new version of the Bayley Scales, the Bayley II, has revised norms and is available from the Psychological Corporation.

team approach should not be underestimated. Pediatric therapists must know their professional limitations. All occupational therapists and physical therapists working with this population should obtain appropriate training on issues related to parental substance abuse. Examples include information on the family dynamics and correlates of substance abuse (e.g., multigenerational use, hostility or maternal depression, withholding of information), the physical signs of adult substance abuse (e.g., extreme fatigue, significant agitation, pinpoint pupils, alcohol on the breath), and the course of addiction and recovery.[11,29] Other team members (e.g., social workers, qualified chemical dependency counselors, specially trained nurses, and psychologists), however, have more in-depth knowledge regarding these issues and the treatment of maternal substance abuse. Therapists should know when and how to refer to other professionals who have expertise in dealing with maternal substance abuse. When the infant displays abnormal developmental findings, pediatric therapists can refer families to developmental pediatricians and dysmorphologists who can diagnose FAS or other developmental delays. In addition, therapists should be familiar with local community resources, including crisis assistance for parents, and be prepared to link families with programs such as therapeutic day care, alcohol and drug hotlines, crisis nursery and respite care, parenting classes and community support groups, and Head Start. One of the most important services pediatric therapists may provide for families affected by substance abuse is linking them with someone in the community who can stay in contact with the child and help advocate for him or her, regardless of the family's ability to function.

Pediatric occupational therapists should not neglect their educational background and clinical training in the mental health field. Occupational therapists specializing in mental health and working in alcohol and drug treatment programs can be a valuable resource for pediatric therapists who are learning to recognize and deal with issues of addiction and recovery. When assessment and interventions take place within the caregiving context, therapists will find their skills in therapeutic communication essential to effective interaction.

The legal and ethical issues in working with this population are complex. Oftentimes it is difficult to sort out what is in the caregiver's and the child's best interest, which may not always be the same. Therapists should know the specific policies and procedures of their agency regarding the identification and documentation of parental substance abuse and understand who within the agency can act as their consultant and back-up. State child abuse laws mandate health care and educational professionals to report suspected cases of child maltreatment. Specific training is helpful in knowing when and how to effectively refer families to child protective agencies.

Pediatric therapists conducting assessments of at-risk infants should know when to recommend therapy for a child affected by prenatal exposure to alcohol or illicit drugs. While many can be unaffected, some of these infants and children have subtle or transient neurological and behavioral deficits. When the child's behavioral state or neuromotor status limits functional performance in motor, social, or language areas, then the infant or child should be referred for therapy (e.g., physical, occupational and/or speech therapy). It is a challenge to decide whether direct therapy intervention is needed, or whether the child and caregiver would be better served by a therapy consultant who provides practical, realistic information to the caregiver on the physical handling and feeding of the child, playing and interacting with the child, and on making the social and physical environment most conducive to developmental progress. In addition to consulting with the family, pediatric therapists should also communicate with multiple professionals such as case managers, public health nurses, and treatment counselors in making decisions about the most appropriate and beneficial methods of service provision. In cases where there are environmental concerns, but not necessarily concerns about the infant's development, the pediatric therapist's role may include periodic monitoring of the child's developmental status and referral to community resources such as therapeutic childcare, parenting classes and Head Start. In summary, the diversity of needs within this population clearly requires therapists to expand their traditional knowledge base to encompass an understanding of addiction and recovery community resources, referral networks, and child welfare policies.

FUTURE DIRECTIONS

Many topics in this area need further study and are of special interest to pediatric therapists. The impact of prenatal drug exposure on the developing child can be quite subtle and may well require the use of sophisticated assessment techniques, such as kinematic analysis of videotaped movements, tests of visual information-processing and recognition memory, and temperament assessment. More studies are needed to carefully examine the quality and diversity of caregiver-infant interactions over time and during situations such as feeding, caregiving, and playing, to further the work of investigators such as Aten,[59] Minkin,[60] and Neuspiel and colleagues.[42]

Clinicians also need empirical data on the efficacy of teaching physical handling and interaction techniques to caregivers raising children who are drug or alcohol affected, as initiated by Schneider and colleagues.[61] Pediatric therapists could investigate the development of sensory processing, sensory integration, and motor skills, as well as attention, memory, learning, and adaptive behavior among infants and children affected by prenatal exposure to drugs or alcohol or both. Research could build on the work discussed by Osborn and colleagues,[19] Coles and Platzman,[28] and in the recent studies of Alessandri and associates,[62] Morse and Cermak,[63] and Adamitis and Lane.[64] Another important area of study involves the optimal type, timing, intensity, and efficacy of early intervention, both home-based and center-based, for children who show fetal alcohol and drug effects.[65]

Investigation into caregiver perceptions about the infant, and what caregivers think about the process of assessment and intervention, may help pediatric therapists better understand these families so that support and information is offered to caregivers at critical times. The use of qualitative methods to explore parents' experiences in raising children during recovery from drugs or alcohol, and during active substance use, may offer real insight to clinicians about which interventions are and are not helpful to families affected by substance abuse.

Just as developmental outcomes result from the interaction between a child and his or her environment, the transactional model also has been influenced and shaped over time by the research and clinical experiences of early childhood professionals. Pediatric therapists can play a key role in contributing to the development of new assessment models and methods for infants and children who are at risk because of prenatal exposure to alcohol or illicit drugs.

REFERENCES

1. Chasnoff IJ, Landress HJ, Barrett ME. The prevalence of illicit-drug or alcohol use during pregnancy and discrepancies in mandatory reporting in Pinellas County, Florida. *N Engl J Med.* 1990;322:1202-1206.

2. Singer LT, Garber R, Kliegman R. Neurobehavioral sequelae of fetal cocaine exposure. *J Pediatr.* 1991;4:667-672.

3. Van Dyke DC, Fox AA. Fetal drug exposure and its possible implications for learning in the preschool and school-age population. *J Learning Disabil.* 1990;3:160-163.

4. Chasnoff IJ, Griffith DR, Freier C, Murray J. Cocaine/polydrug use in pregnancy: two-year follow-up. *Pediatrics.* 1992;89:4-9.

5. Zuckerman B, Bresnahan K. Developmental and behavioral consequences of prenatal drug and alcohol exposure. *Pediatr Clin North Am.* 1991;38:1387-1406.

6. Sameroff AJ, Chandler MJ. Reproductive risk and the continuum of caretaking casualty. In: Horowitz FD, Hetherington M, Scarr-Salapatek S, Siegal S, eds. *Review of Child Development Research.* Vol. 4. Chicago, Ill: University of Chicago Press; 1975:187-244.

7. Greenspan SI, Meisels S. Toward a new vision for the developmental assessment of infants and young children. *Zero to Three.* 1994;14:1-8.

8. Belsky J, Rovine M, Taylor DC. The Pennsylvania Infant and Family Development Project III: the origins of individual differences in mother-infant attachment: maternal and infant contributions. *Child Dev.* 1984;48:182-194.

9. Griffith DR, Freier C. Methodological issues in the assessment of the mother-child interactions of substance-abusing women and their children. In: Kilbey MM, Asghar K, eds. *Methodological Issues in Epidemiological, Prevention, and Treatment Research on Drug-exposed Women and their Children.* Rockville, Md: National Institute on Drug Abuse. 1992; Research Monograph 117:228-247.

10. Reed BG. Developing women-sensitive drug dependence treatment services. *Journal of Psychoactive Drugs.* 1987;19:151-164.

11. Davis SK. Chemical dependency in women: a description of its effects and outcome on adequate parenting (original contribution). *J Substance Abuse Treat.* 1990;7:225-232.

12. Zaichkin J, Houston RF. The drug-exposed mother and infant: a regional center experience. *Neonatal Network.* 1993;12:41-49.

13. Myers BJ, Carmichael Olson H, Kaltenbach K. Cocaine-exposed infants: myths and misunderstandings. *Zero to Three.* 1992;13:1-5.

14. Martin JC. The effects of maternal use of tobacco products or amphetamines on offspring. In: Sonderegger TB, ed. *Perinatal Substance Abuse: Research Findings and Clinical Implications.* Baltimore, Md: The Johns Hopkins University Press; 1992:279-305.

15. *Eighth Special Report to the U.S. Congress on Alcohol and Health.* Washington, DC: US Department of Health and Human Services; 1993.

16. Sokol RJ, Clarren SK. Guidelines for use of terminology describing the impact of prenatal alcohol on the offspring. *Alcoholism Clin Exper Res.* 1989;13:597-598.

17. Streissguth AP, Guinta CT. Symposium on addiction and the family: mental health and health needs of infants and preschool children with fetal alcohol syndrome. *International J Fam Psych.* 1988;9:29-47.

18. Carmichael Olson H. The effects of prenatal alcohol exposure on child development. *Infants and Young Children.* 1994;6:10-25.

19. Osborn JA, Harris SR, Weinberg J. Fetal alcohol syndrome: review of the literature with implications for physical therapists. *Phys Ther.* 1993;73:599-607.

20. Kaltenbach K, Finnegan LP. Prenatal narcotic exposure: perinatal and developmental effects. *Neurotoxicol.* 1989;10:597-604.

21. Wilson GS. Heroin use during pregnancy: clinical studies of long-term effects. In: Sonderegger TB, ed. *Perinatal Substance Abuse: Research Findings and Clinical Implications.* Baltimore, Md: The Johns Hopkins University Press; 1992:224-238.

22. Daltiero SL, Fried PA. The effects of marijuana use on offspring. In: Son-deregger TB, ed. *Perinatal Substance Abuse: Research Findings and Clinical Implications.* Baltimore, Md: The Johns Hopkins University Press; 1992:161-183.

23. Neuspiel DR, Hamel SC. Cocaine and infant behavior (review article). *J Dev Behav Pediatr.* 1991;12:55-64.

24. Mayes LC, Granger RH, Bornstein MH, Zuckerman BS. The problem of prenatal cocaine exposure: a rush to judgment. *JAMA.* 1992;267:406-408.

25. Van Baar AL, Fleury P, Ultee CA. Behavior in the first year after drug dependent pregnancy. *Arch Dis Child.* 1989;64:241-245.

26. Azuma SD, Chasnoff, IJ. Outcome of children prenatally exposed to cocaine and other drugs: a path analysis of three-year data. *Pediatrics.* 1993;92;397-402.

27. Zuckerman B, Frank DA. "Crack kids": Not broken. (commentary) *Pediatrics.* 1992;89:337-339.

28. Coles CD, Platzman KA. Behavioral development in children prenatally exposed to drugs and alcohol. *International J Addict.* 1993;28:1393-1433.

29. Mayes LC. Substance abuse and parenting. In: Bornstein MH, ed. *The Handbook of Parenting.* Hilllsdale, NJ: Erlbaum. In press.

30. Bresnahan K, Brooks C, Zuckerman B. Prenatal cocaine use: impact on infants. *Pediatr Nurs.* 1991;17:123-129.

31. Kaplan-Sanoff M, Parker S, Zuckerman B. Poverty and early childhood development: what do we know, and what should we do? *Infants Young Children.* 1991;4:68-76.

32. Tronick E, Field T, eds. *Maternal Depression and Infant Disturbances: New Directions for Child Development.* San Francisco, Calif: Jossey-Bass; 1986.

33. Lyons-Ruth K, Zoll D, Connell D, Odom R. *Maternal depression as a mediator of the effects of home-based intervention services.* Presented at the biannual meeting of the Society for Research in Child Development. Baltimore, Md; April, 1987.

34. Barnard KE, Kelly JF. Assessment of parent-child interactions. In: Meisels SJ, Shonkoff, JP, eds. *Handbook of Early Childhood Intervention.* Cambridge, Mass: Cambridge University Press; 1990: 278-302.

35. Lewis KD, Bennett B, Schmeder NH. The care of infants menaced by cocaine abuse. *Am J Mat Child Nurs.* 1989;14:324-329.

36. Bayes J. Substance abuse and child abuse: impact of addiction on the child. *Ped Clin N. Am.* 1990;37:881-904.

37. Kelley SJ. Parenting stress and child maltreatment in drug-exposed children. *Child Abuse Neglect.* 1992;16:317-328.

38. Famularo R, Kinscherff R, Fenton T. Parental substance abuse and the nature of child maltreatment. *Child Abuse Neglect.* 1992;16:475-483.

39. Wasserman DR, Leventhal JM. Maltreatment of children born to cocaine-dependent mothers. *AJDC.* 1993;147:1324-1328.

40. Bauman PS, Dougherty FE. Drug-addicted mothers' parenting and their children's development. *International J Addictions.* 1983;18:291-302.

41. Burns K, Chethik L, Burns WJ, Clark R. Dyadic disturbances in cocaine abusing mothers and their infants. *J Clin Psychol.* 1991;47:316-319.

42. Neuspiel DR, Hamel SC, Hochberg E, Greene J, Campbell D. Maternal cocaine use and infant behavior. *Neurotoxicol Teratol.* 1991;13:229-233.

43. Werner EE. Protective factors and individual resilience. In: Meisels SJ, Shonkoff JP, eds. *Handbook of Early Childhood Intervention.* New York, NY: Cambridge University Press; 1990:97-116.

44. Luthar SS, Zigler E. Vulnerability and competence: a review of research on resilience in childhood (theory and review). *Am J Orthopsychiat.* 1991;61:6-21.

45. Bayley N. *Manual for the Bayley Scales of Infant Development.* New York, NY: The Psychological Corporation; 1969.

46. Chandler LS, Andrews M, Swanson M, Larson A. *Movement Assessment of Infants-Screening Test.* Rolling Bay, Wash: Infant Movement Research; 1983.

47. Barnard KE, ed. *Nursing Child Assessment Satellite Training: Parent/Infant Interaction Manual.* Seattle, Wash: Nursing Child Assessment Training Publications; 1980.

48. Chandler LS, Andrews M, Swanson M. *Movement Assessment of Infants.* Rolling Bay, Wash: Infant Movement Research; 1980.

49. Abidin RR. *Parenting Stress Index/Short Form.* Charlottesville, VA: Pediatric Psychology Press; 1990.

50. Farran D, Kasari C, Comfort M, Jay S. Parent/Caregiver Involvement Scale. Chapel Hill, NC: The University of North Carolina at Chapel Hill; 1986.

51. Milner JS. *The Child Abuse Potential Inventory Manual.* 2nd ed. DeKalb, Ill: Psytec Inc; 1986.

52. Bavolek SJ. *Adult-Adolescent Parenting Inventory.* Eau Claire, Wis: Family Development Resources, Inc; 1984.

53. Zeitlin S, Williamson GG, Sczepanski M. *Early Coping Inventory.* Bensenville, Ill: Scholastic Testing Service, Inc.; 1990.

54. Lane SJ. Assessment of infants born after prenatal cocaine exposure. *Dev Disabil Special Interest Newsletter.* 1992;15:2-4.

55. Miller LJ. *Miller Assessment for Preschoolers.* Littleton, Colo: Foundation for Knowledge in Development; 1982.

56. Linder TW. *Transdisciplinary Play-Based Assessment: A Functional Approach to Working with Young Children.* Baltimore, Md: Paul H. Brooks; 1990.

57. Chatoor I, Menvielle E, Getson P, O'Donnell R. *Observational Scale for Mother-Infant Interaction During Feeding.* Washington, DC: Children's Hospital Medical Center; 1988.

58. Achenbach T. *Child Behavior Checklist for Ages 2-3.* Burlington, Vt: Center for Children, Youth and Families, University of Vermont; 1988.

59. Aten MA. *Caregiver-Infant Interactions During Feeding in Infants Prenatally Exposed to Drugs or Alcohol.* Tacoma, Wash: University of Puget Sound; 1994. Unpublished thesis.

60. Minkin JA. *Infant-caregiver play interactions in infants prenatally exposed to drugs or alcohol.* Tacoma, Wash: University of Puget Sound; 1994. Unpublished thesis.

61. Schneider JW, Griffith DR, Chasnoff IR. Infants exposed to cocaine in utero: implications for developmental assessment and intervention. *Infants Young Children.* 1989; 2:25-36.

62. Alessandri SM, Sullivan MW, Imaizumi S, Lewis M. Learning and emotional responsivity in cocaine-exposed infants. *Dev Psych.* 1993;29:989-997.

63. Morse BA, Cermak, SA. Sensory integration in children with fetal alcohol syndrome. *Research Society on Alcoholism.* 1994. Abstract.

64. Adamitis SM, Lane SJ. *Inter-rater Reliability of the Test of Sensory Function in Infants as Used with Infants Prenatally Exposed to Cocaine.* Buffalo, NY: State University of New York at Buffalo; 1992.

65. Carmichael Olson H, Burgess DM. (in press). Early intervention with children prenatally exposed to alcohol and other drugs. In Guralnick M. (Ed.), *The Effectiveness of Early Intervention: Second Generation Research.* Baltimore, Md: Paul H. Brookes.

RESOURCE

Puttkammer CH ed. *Working with Substance-Exposed Children: Strategies for Professionals.* Tucson, AZ: Therapy Skill Builders; 1994.

Issues of Developmental Measurement in Clinical Research and Practice Settings with Children Who Were Prenatally Exposed to Drugs

Ruth Rose-Jacobs
Deborah A. Frank
Elizabeth R. Brown

SUMMARY. Health care providers in clinical and research settings assess the developmental status of increasing numbers of infants and children who were prenatally exposed to drugs. Although assessment of these infants is similar to that of other at-risk infants, limita-

---

Ruth Rose-Jacobs, ScD, PT, is Director of the Infant and Child Development Laboratory, Boston City Hospital, and Adjunct Assistant Professor of Pediatrics, Boston University School of Medicine. Deborah A. Frank, MD, is Director of the Growth and Development Clinic, Boston City Hospital, and Associate Professor of Pediatrics, Boston University School of Medicine. Elizabeth R. Brown, MD, is Director of Neonatology, Boston City Hospital, and Associate Professor of Pediatrics and of Obstetrics and Gynecology, Boston University School of Medicine.

Address correspondence to Ruth Rose-Jacobs, ScD, PT, Old Maternity Building–Second floor, Division of Neonatology, Boston City Hospital, 818 Harrison Avenue, Boston, MA 02118.

This work was supported by grants from: the National Institute on Drug Abuse DA06365 (Dr. Brown) and DA06532 (Dr. Frank); Ronald McDonald Children's Charities (Dr. Frank); and National Institutes of Health Biomedical Research Support Grant (Dr. Rose-Jacobs).

[Haworth co-indexing entry note]: "Issues of Developmental Measurement in Clinical Research and Practice Settings with Children Who Were Prenatally Exposed to Drugs." Rose-Jacobs, Ruth, Deborah A. Frank, and Elizabeth R. Brown. Co-published simultaneously in *Physical & Occupational Therapy in Pediatrics* (The Haworth Press, Inc.) Vol. 16, No. 1/2, 1996, pp. 73-87; and: *Children with Prenatal Drug Exposure* (ed: Lynette S. Chandler, and Shelly J. Lane) The Haworth Press, Inc., 1996, pp. 73-87. Single or multiple copies of this article are available from The Haworth Document Delivery Service [1-800-342-9678, 9:00 a.m. - 5:00 p.m. (EST). E-mail address: getinfo@haworth.com].

© 1996 by The Haworth Press, Inc. All rights reserved.

73

tions and other issues of assessment may be overlooked given societal concerns about drug exposure. In order to meet the evaluation needs of children who were prenatally exposed to drugs, providers must know the limitations associated with the process and instrumentation of assessment, and address the shortcomings of evaluation itself. We review the issues and provide recommendations for change related to measurement; sources of bias; specificity and sensitivity of assessment tools; longitudinal assessment; and multidimensional approaches to assessment. *[Article copies available from The Haworth Document Delivery Service: 1-800-342-9678. E-mail address: getinfo@haworth.com]*

Increasing numbers of infants and children who were prenatally exposed to drugs are assessed yearly within clinical and research settings. Although these infants may exhibit the difficulties and behaviors attributed to at-risk infants with a variety of diagnoses, drug-exposure in particular is frequently surrounded by myths and stereotypes.[1,2] In order to identify objective concerns associated with prenatal drug exposure and determine need for intervention services, physical therapists, occupational therapists, and their colleagues need to document the longitudinal development of these infants and children. Often overlooked in the documentation process are the complexities of assessment itself which may be forgotten temporarily when overshadowed by the concerns of drug-exposure. Perceptions of outcome and longitudinal change frequently can be influenced by the choice of measurement tools.[3,4] The purpose of this article is to elucidate several aspects of measurement from both clinical and research perspectives which are germane to evaluation of the effects of prenatal drug-exposure.

THE PURPOSE OF OUTCOME MEASUREMENT

The usual purpose of developmental assessment within a clinical setting is to identify the child's developmental status and to evaluate the need for intervention.[3,4] It follows that the assessment of infants and children who were prenatally drug-exposed should also identify strengths and deficits. Developmental status identified during evaluation, rather than the mechanism of drug exposure, should be a primary guide for intervention. Maternal drug use is associated with a host of co-morbidities, and developmental outcomes of infants exposed to drugs usually cannot be attributed to the single factor of illicit drug use. The individual but intertwined risk factors associated with substance abuse and poverty are not easily measured.[5] Children of poor inner-city women are at high developmental risk as a result of multiple factors: (1) biologic (e.g., low birthweight), (2) maternal psychosocial (e.g., educational level, affective disorders such as depression), and (3) environmental (e.g., poor nutrition, lack of medical care, violence within the home and community). When these factors are compounded by maternal illicit drug use, risk becomes even greater.[6,7,8] Even illicit drug use is not a singular factor. Women who have abused drugs frequently report using more than one type of illicit drug during pregnancy. Each drug has its own toxicology which is additionally influenced by purity, amount and frequency of use, and timing of use during the pregnancy.[9,10] In addition, pregnant women who use illicit drugs such as cocaine or opiates often also use licit substances with fetal effects, including cigarettes and alcohol. Furthermore, positive HIV status of the child would be a significant factor in the child's developmental course regardless of whether disease transmission was due to maternal drug use.[1]

Within a research setting, large numbers of subjects, careful research design, and complex statistical analyses to evaluate a variety of carefully quantified risk factors must be used before attempting to attribute developmental outcome to a specific drug exposure.[11,12]

EXAMINER KNOWLEDGE OF CHILD HISTORY: AN AREA OF POSSIBLE BIAS

Although clinicians and researchers alike come to assessment with conscious and subconscious biases regarding ultimate developmental outcome,[13] these biases may be particularly influential when dealing with sensitive and highly publicized issues such as maternal drug abuse. For example, clinical perceptions of developmental outcome secondary to maternal drug use during pregnancy may be skewed negatively. Twenty percent of women falsely deny having used illicit drugs during pregnancy.[1,2] As a result, many infants born to mothers who had used illicit drugs during pregnancy may not be identified by maternal history as being drug-exposed. It is reasonable to believe that those infants who were drug-exposed, but not identified as such by maternal history, would be less likely to be referred for developmental assessment or services unless there were other presenting concerns. In addition, prenatally exposed infants who are referred are more likely to be a subset of infants whose development is influenced by a constellation of negative risk factors, all of which might be associated with a final common neurologic pathway. Subsequently, clinicians who assess and treat at-risk infants may relate prenatal drug exposure to a clinical picture that represents only the most compromised subset of infants.

Few studies have directly evaluated examiner bias related to infant drug exposure. One study, however, examined the influence of physical therapists' previous knowledge of medical history on assessments of at-risk infants using the Movement Assessment of Infants.[14] After viewing a videotaped assessment of both a high-risk and a low-risk infant, four groups of therapists, each with different information regarding the infants' medical history, scored the assessments. The greatest discrepancy in scores, i.e., highest false-positive identification, occurred in ratings from the group of therapists who assessed the low-risk infant they believed to have a high-risk history. Given this demonstration of bias based on history, clinicians should weigh the positive and negative implications of obtaining extensive infant histories prior to assessment of at-risk infants. Examiners in a research setting should be masked to children's group assignment.[13,14]

Although it is obvious that therapists should be comfortable interacting with the variety of caretakers who may accompany children, the issue of being able to relate comfortably to caretakers who may have used drugs is particularly important. In either clinical or research settings, physical therapists and occupational therapists should consider their own thoughts and biases about drug abuse and determine how such feelings might influence assessments and interactions with the family. Caretakers may change over time and might include a mother who is currently using drugs or a mother who has made varying levels of progress within a drug treatment program. If practice is to be family-centered, pediatric therapists should educate themselves on issues of adult addiction and work closely with social workers and other mental health professionals to facilitate referrals for family services and support as necessary. In order to maintain professional objectivity and avoid burnout, clinicians and researchers who work extensively with high-risk children in families with substance abuse problems should have access to periodic and professionally-led support meetings for providers.

ASSESSMENT CONCERNS ASSOCIATED WITH MEASUREMENT TOOLS

An important use of normed and standardized assessments is the identification of children's abilities in relation to similar-age peers.[4] Infants who were prenatally drug-exposed, like other at-risk infants, require long term follow-up to determine their ongoing developmental trajectory in relationship to peers. Instrument characteristics or *sole* use of these normed and standardized assessments with at-risk infants could, however, significantly limit evaluation findings.[3] Only comprehensive repeated assessments can determine whether possible deviations or subtle nuances might be of developmental significance. To address some assessment concerns associated with these infants, three areas of particular concern will be discussed: (1) sensitivity and specificity of assessment tools, (2) longitudinal discontinuities of performance domains across assessment tools, and (3) the limited scope of developmental domains associated with specific assessment tools.

Sensitivity and Specificity of Assessment Tools

Evidence exists that some assessment tools may not be sensitive enough to identify subtle but important signs of developmental differences in a variety of at-risk groups. At-risk infants such as those who were born preterm,[15,16] low birth weight,[17] or with in-utero exposure to drugs,[11,18] are reported to score within normal limits on standardized assessments despite examiner concerns about the quality of infant performance. Clinicians often supplement results of norm-referenced assessments with anecdotal descriptions of an individual's qualitative performance, a practice that is often time consuming and subjective. Researchers, who evaluate group data and often rely heavily on the summary scores of developmental indexes, may be more affected by this measurement limitation. Study outcomes, therefore, may be influenced by the sensitivity of the assessment instruments.

Infants who were drug-exposed have been inadequately studied because of multiple methodologic difficulties associated with research on this population. Until more is known about these infants, inferences about assessment sensitivity and specificity from research on other types of at-risk infants cautiously could be used to anticipate concerns about assessment tools when used with infants who were drug-exposed. Studies comparing infants born preterm or fullterm reported both groups to have developmental index scores on the Bayley Scales of Infant Development (BSID) that were within normal limits. After BSID items were grouped and further analyzed, however, infants born preterm were less likely to pass certain groups of items than infants born at term.[15,19] A review of developmental studies comparing infants who were opioid-exposed and infants who were non-drug-exposed reported that summative scores (such as the developmental indexes of the BSID) show only weak discrimination between the two groups. Qualitative descriptors were often better measures of discrimination than rates of skill acquisition.[20] Because the

Bayley Scales have recently been revised and renormed, new studies are needed to assess their sensitivity and specificity.[21]

Chasnoff and colleagues reported that two 24-month-old infant groups (cocaine, marijuana and/or alcohol-exposed; and marijuana and/or alcohol but not cocaine-exposed) had greater proportions of BSID scores more than two standard deviations below the mean as compared to an unexposed control group.[22] Mean BSID scores of the three groups, however, did not differ significantly. At the 3-year data point the same research group identified a hypothesized path model of effect whereby prenatal substance exposure indirectly affected Stanford-Binet scores through relationships with home environment, head circumference, and behavior.[23] Identification of infant group differences may be influenced by the sensitivity and specificity of assessment tools, method of summarizing test results, and ages of children at the time of assessment.

It is obvious that follow-up clinical and research assessments of infants who were drug-exposed should be planned carefully to measure specific areas of hypothesized deficit. New normed and standardized primary assessment tools should also be developed to address subtle areas of concern.[20] In the meantime, a screening tool which may be useful for children who were prenatally exposed to drugs is the Miller Assessment for Preschoolers (MAP).[24] The MAP tests sensory, motor, and cognitive (verbal and non-verbal) areas of development. Because it was developed to identify children with mild to moderate delays, the MAP is thought to be most useful in identifying mildly delayed or "pre-learning-disabled" children.[25] Some children who were prenatally exposed to drugs may fall within this category.

Additional advances in the evaluation of at-risk children, including children who were prenatally exposed to drugs, also could be made by the development of supplemental measures of assessment. These measures could help to quantify heretofore non-quantified aspects of observed behavior during testing. An ancillary tool that was recently developed to augment the known strengths of a "gold standard" assessment, is the Performance Qualifying Scale (PQS) for use with the Bayley Scales of Infant Development.[26] The PQS (Figure 1), developed by Rose-Jacobs and colleagues, can be used to improve documentation of examiners' qualitative observations during administration of the Bayley Scales of Infant Development (BSID) and the newly revised Bayley II.[21] The PQS is a five-point scoring system that refines the pass/fail BSID scoring and objectifies examiner perceptions of the quality of infant performance on each item as follows: 5 = consistent pass; 4 = inconsistent pass; 3 = pass achieved via accidental, alternative, or qualitatively inappropriate means; 2 = partial but unsuccessful attempt; 1 = no attempt. An example of a pass qualified as "3" would be an infant who manages to roll from supine to prone without the usual dissociation between shoulder and pelvic girdles. For analytic purposes, the PQS scores for each BSID item can be grouped and averaged within five developmental subdomains (cognitive, language, social, fine motor, gross motor),[27] or defined by the categories of the Bayley II. In this manner, the PQS identifies the average quality of performance within each of five domains which would not otherwise be systematically documented. The PQS has an average inter-rater reliability of .89 (range of .81 to 1.00) agreement.[26]

An initial validity study evaluated the PQS as a complement to the BSID in discriminating high and low risk infants in a sample of 52 fullterm, 6-month-old inner-city infants whose mothers had *not* used cocaine or opiates as documented by urine and meconium assays.[27] Fine motor PQS scores significantly differentiated the most impoverished infants (those mothers receiving AFDC) within an already low socioeconomic sample. In contrast, MDI and PDI scores from the BSID failed to discriminate between these groups. Further study is needed to determine the validity of the PQS for discriminating between infants of similar SES backgrounds who are drug-exposed and non-drug-exposed, controlling for SES.

Longitudinal Measurement: Significance and Concerns

Longitudinal measurement of developmental status is of particular importance with infants who were prenatally exposed to drugs. Without multi-

FIGURE 1. Performance Qualifying Scale (PQS) for Use with the Bayley Scales of Infant Development

5 = COMPLETE AND CONSISTENT RESPONSE: Easily and consistently *completes* item in a manner appropriate for the level of the item. (Pass by BSID criteria)

4 = COMPLETE BUT INCONSISTENT RESPONSE: *Completes* item with difficulty or inconsistency. May be able to complete the item only one direction. (Pass by BSID criteria)

3 = COMPLETES CRITERIA OF ITEM BY ACCIDENT OR USE OF *ALTERNATIVE* MEANS: Item completion is seemingly by chance, with abnormal movement patterns, or in an otherwise alternative manner. (Pass by BSID criteria)
- -
2 = PARTIAL RESPONSE: Child attempts item but unable to pass criteria. (Fail by BSID criteria)

1 = NO RESPONSE: Child does not attempt the presented item. (Fail by BSID criteria)

ple assessments over time it is difficult to interpret the significance of early neuromotor signs. If testing is restricted to infancy, it is difficult to identify and interpret developmental problems which might appear only when more complex functional and cognitive demands can be placed on an older child.[4] Only a few studies have followed children who were drug-exposed into middle childhood.[20,28,29] Information varies by type of drug exposure, and little objective information is known about these children's long term developmental outcome. Outcomes after several years of children who experienced neonatal heroin withdrawal, demonstrated transient dystonia, participated in intervention programs, or grew up in supportive environments are but three significant areas needing further investigation.

Measurement over a period of years brings unique challenges to the assessment process. As age increases, different developmental abilities are highlighted, and different assessment tools are used. One particular problem of longitudinal assessment with standardized assessment tools is discontinuity of developmental domains across assessment tools. To illustrate this important problem, three frequently used assessments for young drug-exposed and other at-risk infants, the Neonatal Behavioral Assessment Scale (NBAS),[30] Movement Assessment of Infants (MAI),[31] and the Bayley Scales of Infant Development (BSID) and the newly revised Bayley II[21] will be discussed. The Bayley II will be addressed in both forms because some clinical facilities and current longitudinal research studies are still using the older edition of the assessment.

All three assessments were developed to assess key skills and behaviors within specific age spans. The primary constructs of the NBAS relate to neurophysiology, neurobehavior, and neurodevelopment during the first month of life; the MAI reflects neurophysiology and neurodevelopment with risk scores at 4 and 8 months of age; and the BSID and Bayley II assess neurodevelopment from birth to two and three years of age within the context of cognitive, motor, and behavioral skill acquisition. Although the NBAS, MAI, and BSID assess overlapping aspects of motor development, each is based on a different theoretical framework and each has different strengths. Both the NBAS and the MAI can be used to assess muscle tone, reflexes, and volitional movement. The BSID (and Bayley II) assesses acquisition of motor tasks (rather than neuromotor development) with some gradation of specific abilities across age depending on the number of items testing particular tasks. Problems of muscle tone (an area of concern for infants who were exposed to drugs) are, therefore, recorded on the NBAS, MAI, and Behavior Record Scale (BRS) of the Bayley II, but are not adequately reflected on the BSID. The Infant Behavior Record

(IBR) of the BSID rates body tension, a measure which differs from the physiologic conceptualization of muscle tone.

The problem of discontinuity of developmental domains across assessment instruments will be further illustrated by a composite at-risk infant who presents many of the symptoms hypothesized to be associated with drug exposure. An NBAS assessment on this hypothetical infant could document motoric and behavioral immaturities (e.g., immature reflexes, limited head control, poor habituation to extraneous stimuli, limited interactions with the assessor). In addition, the NBAS supplementary items could document the infant's high-cost-of-attention behaviors (rapid breathing, palor, spitting up), hyper- and/or hypotonicity, significant difficulties in responding to people and objects, and need for considerable examiner assistance (swaddling, rocking, examiner voice modulation). At the four-month follow-up assessment of this hypothetical infant, the MAI could document the infant's level of risk for significant neuromotor problems. Specific items might document hypo- and/or hypertonicity, immature reflexes and reactions, and immature and/or concerning volitional movement (e.g., quality of head control, truncal control in supported postures, absence or quality of reaching). The MAI would not document the infant's possible difficulties in quality of interactions with the examiner in response to stimuli, or possible need for continual examiner structuring during the testing which might have been identified in the neonatal period on the NBAS. In later infancy, it is reasonable to expect that the hypothetical infant (like most at-risk infants) might have average BSID standard (100 ± 16) scores. Alone the MDI and PDI scores on the BSID would not indicate whether level and quality of specific subdomains (cognitive, language, social, fine motor, and gross motor) were age-appropriate. Global scores would not indicate whether remnants of earlier problems associated with immature reflexes, delayed reaching at 4 months, poor truncal control, and problems with interactions and over-reactivity to stimulation might continue to be present. Given the earlier description of follow-up assessment with available standardized tools, testing with parallel items or groups of items is needed which could measure connected constructs of development in at-risk infants over an extended range of ages. To accomplish this goal, additional methods of longitudinal developmental analysis may need to be identified and used in clinical and research settings.

Measurement, although primarily associated with an initial assessment of a child, is also important to quantify progress while a child is participating in an intervention program. Progress towards short-term goals should be measured in an objective manner, using more structured reporting rather than an open narrative note. Two problems hinder the ability to use such an approach to documentation: (1) gains associated with therapeutic goals are often not in areas easily measured by conventional assessment tools, and (2) gains might occur in smaller increments of change than can be sensed by those tools.

One approach to the assessment of change resulting from therapeutic intervention is goal attainment scaling (GAS). GAS is an individualized criterion-referenced method of measuring change.[32] GAS has been successfully used with children[33] who have motor delay and could easily be used with those who were exposed to drugs. Use of GAS might document subtle and functional changes relevant to specific goals of intervention. Following the thorough evaluation of a child, a therapist using GAS identifies short-term goal(s) and five measurable levels of potential goal attainment represented by a scale of -2 to $+2$ for each therapeutic objective. Of concern, however, is possible bias associated with the same therapist creating the goals, treating the child, and measuring progress towards the goals. As a result, we advise that multiple therapists who have attained previous interrater reliability cooperate in the use of the GAS.

Scope: Importance of Multidimensional Approaches to Measurement

Subtle early sensorimotor and neurologic problems in at-risk infants, including infants exposed in-utero to drugs, have been postulated to be precursors to later developmental difficulties not confined necessarily to motor development.[34] Developmental concerns may appear to be diffuse and uneven *within* as well as *across* traditional subdomains, particularly because longitudinal development can be nonlinear in addition to being influenced by the interaction of individual biology and the environment.[18,35,36,37,38] How well these types of concerns can be measured is dependent on the assessment approach and choice of specific assessment tools to adequately assess areas of observed and hypothesized concern.[39] The following discussion will explore the belief that a comprehensive evaluation approach should address developmental concerns at a variety of functional levels.[40] Because physical therapists and occupational therapists are particularly interested in neuromotor output, one of the earliest and most observable areas in young infants, discussion will focus on areas related to motor function.

Early neuromotor signs, such as tremors or variations in muscle tone, and behaviors such as decreased consolability or hyper- or hypo-responsiveness to stimuli are concerns often attributed to young infants who are drug-exposed, particularly to opiates.[34] By the end of a few months these neuromotor signs often decrease significantly and neurobehavioral and neurodevelopmental subtle signs rather than overt abnormalities may persist.[1,41] The original neuromotor concerns might, therefore, be characterized as transient (e.g., transient dystonia) and of questionable long-term importance. Longitudinal patterns of strengths and difficulties *may* be more easily traced, however, when conceptualized and assessed as belonging to global functional categories, such as perceptual-, or behavioral-motor, rather than the singular category of motor, or even the dual categories of fine and gross motor.[42,43] Clinicians and researchers should also evaluate motor output simultaneously within multiple and intercorrelated (but not interchangeable) perspectives by using, for example, assessment tools which specifically address areas such as neuromotor, sensory processing, attention, and motor skill and/or control. Use of this more comprehensive approach to infant neurodevelopmental assessment could be one means of relating early subtle developmental concerns to later deficits when areas such as sensorimotor processing or perception can be more directly assessed.

The traditional practice of dividing overall development into conventional subdomains such as cognition, language, social, and gross and fine motor may be misleading for drug-exposed and other types of at-risk infants. Although some infants with early neuromotor problems apparently "recover" from transient dystonia, later school and cognitive issues may also still exist. These later-recognized problems range from concerns about attention and visual-motor integration to concerns about overt learning disabilities.[35,36,44] Evidence suggests that transient dystonia might be a marker for later behavioral problems including hyperactivity, impulsivity, and cognitive and speech delays.[37,45] Comprehensive, multidimensional, and sometimes alternative approaches to standardized assessment of infants who were exposed to drugs may clarify apparent discontinuities. Assessment approaches and specific assessment tools could be drawn from those used by a variety of disciplines depending on the particular educational background of clinicians and the physical resources within a facility. Evaluative approaches which include play, perceptual paradigms, kinematics, mother-child interaction paradigms, and behavioral checklists are but a few means of supplementing standardized or traditional physical therapy and occupational therapy measures, and these approaches may be of particular importance for children who were drug-exposed.[46,47] The interdisciplinary use of some of these approaches to assessment could help to bridge the gap between traditional assessments, bring particularly productive insights to the evaluation of the specific child, and develop broader perspectives for those professionals involved in the assessment process.[48]

CONCLUSION

If the outcomes of longitudinal research and clinical practice are to meet the challenge of assessing infants and children who were prenatally drug-exposed, then therapists need to be aware of important issues related to assessment and encouraged to address some of the limitations associated with the process and current instrumentation. Physical therapists and occupational therapists need to evaluate possible sources of bias which could be problematic when assessing infants and children who were drug-exposed. Primary and ancillary assessment instruments need to be developed and adequately assessed to determine reliability, validity, sensitivity, and specificity. Optimally, new assessment instruments need to quantify significant but heretofore undocumented areas of concern at particular ages and across the developmental course. Simultaneously, areas of assessment may need to be conceptually re-evaluated and opportunities for interdisciplinary assessment and cooperation improved.

REFERENCES

1. Brown ER, Zuckerman B. The infant of drug-abusing mothers. *Pediatric Annals.* 1991;20:555-563.
2. Frank DF, Bresnahan K, Zuckerman BS. Maternal cocaine use: Impact on child health and development. *Advances in Pediatrics.* 1993;40:65-99.
3. McCune L, Kalmanson B, Fleck M, Glazewski B, Sillari J. An interdisciplinary model of infant assessment. In: Meisels S, Shonkoff J eds. *Handbook of Early Childhood Interventions.* New York, NY: Cambridge University Press; 1990:246-277.
4. Cicchetti D, Wagner S. Alternative assessment strategies for the evaluation of infants and toddlers: An organizational perspective. In: Meisels S, Shonkoff J eds. *Handbook of Early Childhood Intervention.* New York, NY: Cambridge University Press; 1990:246-277.
5. Johnson HL, Glassman MB, Fiks KB, Rosen TS. Path analysis of variables affecting 36-month outcome in a population of multi-risk children. *Infant Behavior and Development.* 1987;10:451-465.
6. Zuckerman BS, Frank DA. "Crack kids": Not broken. *Pediatrics.* 1992; 89:337-339.
7. Johnson HL, Rosen TS. Mother-infant interaction in a multirisk population. *Amer J Orthopsychiat.* 1990;60:281-288.
8. Regan DO, Ehrlich SM, Finnegan LP. Infants of drug addicts: At risk for child abuse, neglect, and placement in foster care. *Neurotoxicology and Teratology.* 1987;9:315-319.
9. Szeto HH. Maternal-fetal pharmacokinetics and fetal dose-response relationship. *Annals of the New York Academy of Sciences.* 1989;562:42-55.
10. Mayes LC, Granger RH, Bornstein MH, Zuckerman B. The problem of prenatal cocaine exposure. *JAMA.* 1992;267:406-408.
11. Jacobson J. Discussion: Measurement of drug-induced physical and behavioral delays and abnormalities—A general framework. *NIDA Monograph Series.* 1991;114:182-186.

12. Johnson SB. Methodological considerations in pediatric behavioral research: Measurement. *Developmental and Behavioral Pediatr.* 1991;12:361-369.

13. Bartlett D, Piper MC. Neuromotor development of preterm infants through the first year of life: Implications for physical and occupational therapists. *Physical & Occupational Therapy in Pediatr.* 1993;12:(4):37-55.

14. Ashton B, Piper MC, Warren S, Stewin L, Byrne P. Influence of medical history on assessment of at-risk infants. *Dev Med Child Neurol.* 1991;33:412-418.

15. Ross G. Use of the Bayley Scales to characterize abilities of premature infants. *Child Dev.* 1985;56:835-842.

16. Aylward GP, Verhulst SJ, Bell S. The early neuropsychologic optimality rating scale (ENORS-9): A new developmental follow-up technique. *J Dev Behav Pediatr.* 1988;9:140-146.

17. Vo D, Burrows E, Beeghly M. "The Qualifier Coding System for Toddlers (QCS-T): A Qualitative Assessment of Two Year Olds." Presented at the National Training Institute of the National Center for Clinical Infant Programs. Washington, DC: Dec 1989.

18. Volpe JJ. Effects of cocaine on the fetus. *NEJ Med.* 1992;327(6):399-407.

19. Rose-Jacobs R. Preterm infant abilities as characterized by the Bayley Scales of Infant Development. *Pediatr Phys Ther.* 1990;3(4):210.

20. Hans SL. Following drug-exposed infants into middle childhood: Challenges to researchers. *NIDA Research Monogr.* 1991;114:310-322.

21. Bayley N. *Bayley Scales of Infant Development I and II.* New York, NY: The Psychological Corporation; 1969, 1993.

22. Chasnoff IJ, Griffith DR, Freier C, Murray J. Cocaine/polydrug use in pregnancy: Two-year Follow-up. *Pediatr.* 1992;89:284-289.

23. Azuma SD, Chasnoff IJ. Outcome of children prenatally exposed to cocaine and other drugs: A path analysis of three-year data. *Pediatr.* 1993; 92:396-402.

24. Miller LJ. *Miller Assessment for Preschoolers.* San Antonio, TX: The Psychological Corporation; 1992.

25. Linder T. Miller Assessment for Preschoolers. In: Keyser DJ, Sweetland RC eds. *Test Critiques* Volume 1. Kansas City, MO: Test Corporation of America; 1985:443-454.

26. Rose-Jacobs R, Beeghly M, Tronick EZ, Brown R, Cabral H, Frank DA. The Performance Qualifying Scale (PQS) for use with the Bayley Scales of Infant Development. *Pediatr Res.* 1993;35:26A.

27. Reuter J, Staccin T, and Craig P. *The Kent Scoring Adaptation of the Bayley Scales of Infant Development.* Kent, OH: Kent Development Metrics; 1981.

28. Barr H, Streissguth AP, Darby B, Sampson P. Prenatal exposure to alcohol, caffeine, tobacco, and aspirin: Effects on fine and gross motor performance in 4-year-old children. *Dev Psychol.* 1990;26:339-348.

29. Fried PA, Watkinson B. 36 and 48-month neurobehavioral follow-up of children prenatally exposed to marijuana, cigarettes, and alcohol. *Dev Behav Pediatr.* 1990;11:49-58.

30. Brazelton TB. *Neonatal Behavioral Assessment Scale*, 2nd ed. Philadelphia, PA: Lippincott; 1984.

31. Chandler LS, Andrews MS, Swanson MW. *Movement Assessment of Infants: A Manual*. Rolling Bay, WA: Authors; 1980.

32. Palisano RJ, Haley SM, Brown DA. Goal attainment scaling as a measure of change in infants with motor delays. *Phys Ther.* 1992;72:432-437.

33. Stephens TE, Haley SM. Comparison of two methods for determining change in motorically handicapped children. *Physical & Occupational Therapy in Pediatrics.* 1991;11(1):1-17.

34. Hans SL, Marcus J, Jeremy RJ, Auerbach JG. Neurobehavioral development of children exposed in utero to opiate drugs. In: Yanai J ed. *Neurobehavioral Teratology*. Amsterdam: Elsevier; 1984;249-273.

35. Ross G, Lipper EG, Auld PA. Consistency and change in the development of premature infants weighing less than 1,501 grams at birth. *Pediatr.* 1985;76:885-891.

36. Siegel L. Infants tests as predictors of cognitive and language development at two years. *Child. Dev.* 1981;52:545-557.

37. Vohr BR, Garcia Coll CT. Neurodevelopmental and school preformance of very low-birth-weight infants: A seven year longitudinal study. *Pediatr.* 1985;76:345-350.

38. Sameroff AJ, Chandler MJ. Reproductive risk and the continuum of caretaking casualty. In: Horowitz FD, Hetherington EM, Scarr-Salapatek S, Siegel GM eds. *Review of Child Development Research*: vol. 4. Chicago, IL: University of Chicago Press; 1975.

39. Hauser-Cram P, Shonkoff J. Rethinking the assessment of child focused outcomes. In: Weiss H, Jacobs F eds. *Evaluating Family Programs*. Hawthorne, NY: Hendrick Publishing; 1988.

40. Campbell SK. Measurement of motor performance in cerebral palsy. In: Forssberg H, Hirshberg H eds. *Movement Disorders in Children*. New York, NY: Karger; 1991;264-271.

41. Brown ER, Cole J, Parker S, Coulter D, Corwin M, Abozgyne K. Treatment of newborn narcotic abstinence to normalize infant behavior. *Pediatr Res.* 1989;25:12A.

42. von Hofsten C. Development of manual actions from a perceptual perspective. In: Forssberg H, Hirshberg H eds. *Movement Disorders in Children*. New York, NY: Karger; 1991:113-123.

43. Jacobson SW, Jacobson JJ, Sokol RJ, Martier SS, Ager JW. Prenatal alcohol exposure and infant information processing ability: *Child Dev.* 199;64:1806-1721.

44. O'Brien VO, Cermak SA, Murray EA. The relationship between visual-perceptual motor abilities and clumsiness in children with and without learning disabilities. *Am J Occup Ther.* 1988; 42:359-363.

45. Saigal S, Rosenbaum P, Szatmari P, Campbell D. Learning disabilities and school problems in a regional cohort of extremely low birthweight children: A comparison with term controls. *Dev Behav Pediatr.* 1991;12:294-300.

46. Robins LN, Mills JL. Effects of in utero exposure to street drugs. *Amer J Pub Health.* 1993;83(Supplement)1-32.

47. Tronick EZ, Beeghly M, Fetters L, Weinberg K. New methodologies for evaluating residual brain damage in infants exposed to drugs of abuse: Objective methods for describing movement, facial expressions, and communication behaviors. *NIDA Research Monograph.* 1991;114:262-290.

48. Kenny TJ, Holden EW, Santilli L. The meaning of measures: Pitfalls in behavioral and development research. *Dev Behav Pediatr.* 1991;12(6):355-360.

Motor Behavior in Children Exposed Prenatally to Drugs

Mary P. Grattan
Sydney L. Hans

SUMMARY. The motor behavior of 35 children with a documented history of prenatal exposure to opioid drugs and 41 comparison children with no history of prenatal substance exposure was assessed from birth to approximately ten years of age using a clinical neurological examination and electronically quantified tests of motor steadiness. There were no opioid exposure effects on the skills assessed by the clinical neurological examination. An interaction was found between prenatal opioid-exposure and age of child on the motor steadiness tasks with deficits related to opioid exposure only observable before the tenth birthday. In discussion emphasis is placed on the range of motor skills in opioid-exposed children and on implications for clinical practice. *[Article copies available from The Haworth Document Delivery Service: 1-800-342-9678. E-mail address: getinfo@haworth.com]*

In recent years considerable concern has been directed toward the developmental outcome of children whose mothers use drugs of abuse during pregnancy. This concern has led at times to forecasts of dire outcomes for children who are prenatally exposed to drugs (The crack children, *Newsweek*, February 1990; Innocent Victims, *Time*, 1991), even though

Mary P. Grattan, PhD, PT, and Sydney L. Hans are affiliated with the Department of Psychiatry at The University of Chicago.
Address correspondence to Sydney L. Hans, Department of Psychiatry, MC3077, The University of Chicago, 5841 South Maryland Avenue, Chicago, IL 60637.

[Haworth co-indexing entry note]: "Motor Behavior in Children Exposed Prenatally to Drugs." Grattan, Mary P., and Sydney L. Hans. Co-published simultaneously in *Physical & Occupational Therapy in Pediatrics* (The Haworth Press, Inc.) Vol. 16, No. 1/2, 1996, pp. 89-109; and: *Children with Prenatal Drug Exposure* (ed: Lynette S. Chandler, and Shelly J. Lane) The Haworth Press, Inc., 1996, pp. 89-109. Single or multiple copies of this article are available from The Haworth Document Delivery Service [1-800-342-9678, 9:00 a.m. - 5:00 p.m. (EST). E-mail address: getinfo@haworth.com].

© 1996 by The Haworth Press, Inc. All rights reserved.   *89*

the small number of carefully conducted research studies assessing the development of prenatally exposed children past the earliest months of infancy report few behavioral problems attributable to prenatal exposure.[1]

Behavioral teratology, the scientific discipline devoted to the study of the postnatal behavioral effects of prenatal exposure to drugs, is a relatively young field.[2] Most behavioral teratology research has been conducted in laboratories in which potentially harmful agents are administered to pregnant animals under carefully controlled conditions.[3] Studies with human populations have been far fewer in number, and for obvious reasons, have employed non-experimental research paradigms.[4] Studies in behavioral teratology with human populations present numerous methodological challenges including accurate assessment of patterns of maternal drug use, selection of appropriate comparison populations, and scrutiny of factors that might be confounded with maternal drug use. Human studies also face the challenge of identifying those neurobehavioral measures most likely to be sensitive to teratologic effects.[4]

Measures of motor behavior have often been adopted as outcome measures in human behavioral teratology studies and offer certain advantages over assessments of intelligence and other complex behavior patterns such as play and language. Motor outcomes can be assessed at all ages, including the first days after birth. Motor behavior is less likely than other complex behavioral outcomes such as language to be adversely influenced by variations in childrearing patterns that in American culture are associated with social class. Additionally, measures of motor behavior have been shown to be sensitive to other types of prenatal insult and pregnancy complications, including preterm delivery.[5-6]

In this paper, we will consider the effects on motor behavior of prenatal exposure to opioid drugs. We will do so first by reviewing the existing literature on motor behavior of children exposed to opioids and then present data from the first long-term follow-up of motor behavior in children exposed in utero to opioids.

Review of Existing Literature

Abuse of opioid drugs, those substances that pharmacologically are related to morphine, is a long-standing social problem in the United States.[7] In the United States most opioid abuse involves illicit heroin, intravenously injected, and sometimes used in combination with cocaine. Recently, pure, smokable forms of heroin have also begun to be available.[8]

Since the mid-1970s, chronic heroin addicts who seek treatment in the United States have often been admitted to government- and privately-funded methadone maintenance programs where they receive free daily oral doses of methadone, a synthetic opioid.[9] Methadone has effects similar to, but longer lasting than, those of heroin, thus making methadone better suited for treatment programs in which medication is administered on a once-daily basis. Methadone is generally dispensed in a clinic setting that may also provide a variety of social services and medical supervision to its clients. In general, people maintained on methadone lead more stable lives than they did as heroin addicts and are assured of better pharmacological control of their habits.

Research literature on the effects of prenatal heroin and methadone exposure in children dates back twenty years. Opioid drugs easily cross the placenta[10] and have effects on the fetus that can be clearly observed during the neonatal period. Clinically, a great deal of concern has been focused on the clear pattern of neonatal abstinence demonstrated by infants in the days following birth.[11-12] Paralleling adult narcotics withdrawal, the medical signs of neonatal abstinence include high fever, sweating, lacrimation, sleeplessness, rapid respiration, vomiting, and diarrhea. A number of studies have explored motor behavior during abstinence by comparing newborns who were opioid-exposed with carefully selected unexposed newborns using the Neonatal Behavioral Assessment Scale.[13] Consistently these studies have reported that, during withdrawal, neonates are hypertonic, jerky, and tremulous in their movements.[14-23] Hypertonicity has also been documented using electromyography.[24]

Relatively little is known about the long-term effects of prenatal opioid exposure on motor behavior. A few animal studies support the notion that prenatal exposure to opioids may alter post-natal motoric development. There have been reports of delayed motor development in rats,[25-26] impaired motor coordination and gait in mice,[27] and alterations in neuromuscular performance in chicks.[28]

In four studies, the acquisition of motor milestones by children who were opioid-exposed has been tracked longitudinally from birth into the second year of life using the Psychomotor Development Index (PDI) from the Bayley Scales of Infant Development.[29] The PDI is a developmental quotient (DQ) that has been normed (like intelligence quotients) so that average performance for age results in a score of 100 and the standard deviation for the population is 16. Table 1 summarizes the mean Bayley PDI scores of the opioid and comparison infants reported in the four studies. In three of these studies, investigators supplemented the PDI with additional measures of motor behavior.

In their study of children in Detroit, Strauss and colleagues[30] compared the PDI scores of methadone-exposed and unexposed infants at three, six, and twelve months of age. Those who were methadone-exposed had poor-

TABLE 1. Bayley PDI Scores in Published Studies of Infants Exposed to Opioids

Study	Age in Months							
	3	4	6	8	9	12	18	24
Detroit[30]								
Opioid	119		109			103*		
Comparison	117		112			110		
Houston[31]								
Methadone					90*			
Heroin					92			
Comparison					99			
New York[32-33]								
Opioid			101			95*	93*	99*
Comparison			105			103	105	108
Chicago[35]								
Opioid		117		112		108	106	101*
Comparison		122		112		110	110	109

* Opioid group differs significantly from comparison group

er scores than the unexposed infants at the twelve-month assessment. In addition, the methadone-exposed, but not the unexposed infants showed a significant drop in PDI scores over the first year of life.

In their Houston sample, Wilson, Desmond, and Wait[31] assessed infants who were methadone-exposed, heroin-exposed, and unexposed at 9 months of age and found significantly poorer PDI scores in the methadone group compared to the unexposed group. In addition to using the developmental quotients from the Bayley Scales, this research group also reported data from the Bayley Infant Behavior Record (IBR), a set of summary clinical rating scales designed to follow the Bayley test items in order to capture qualitative aspects of the infant's behavior. In the Houston sample, the methadone-exposed group had poorer average IBR ratings of fine motor coordination than the unexposed children.

In a study of children in New York City, Rosen, Johnson and colleagues[32-33] reported that prenatal methadone exposure was related to delays in motoric development at 12, 18, and 24 months of age on the Bayley Scales of Infant Development. These researchers also administered a neurological examination to their sample and observed an increased incidence of neurological signs at 18- and 24-months including tone and coordination abnormalities and abnormal ocular findings (such as nystagmus and strabismus). At 36 months of age,[34] a higher incidence of suspect or abnormal neurological findings was observed in the methadone-exposed group (32%) compared to unexposed children (13%).

In a study of children in Chicago, Hans, Marcus and colleagues[35] reported Bayley data on infants from 4, 8, 12, 18, and 24 months of age and found that methadone exposure resulted in statistically significant delays only at 24 months. Examining the Bayley IBR ratings of motoric functioning, the investigators found a pattern of abnormal development in virtually all children in the methadone-exposed group at 4 months that included poor fine and gross motor coordination, high tension, and high activity level.[36-37] In the same sample at 24 months of age, the investigators also reported poorer clinical ratings of fine and gross motor coordination in the methadone-exposed group.[38] These differences were apparent even after controlling for other medical and social risk factors.

Taken together, these four studies suggest that there may be post-neonatal motor delays or poorer coordination in infants exposed prenatally to opioid drugs. Each of the four studies found significant differences in acquisition of motor milestones at one or more ages related to opioid exposure. The three studies that employed assessments of motor functioning during infancy in addition to developmental quotients all found significant differences in motor functioning related to opioid exposure. Finally, in the three samples that included repeated developmental assessments, discrepancies in motor performance between opioid-exposed and unexposed groups increased with age during infancy, although none of the studies reported data past the age of 36 months. Despite the consistency of findings across the studies, however, it should be noted that the mean scores of the infants' psychomotor developmental quotients during infancy remained within normal limits in each of the four studies. Data were not reported in a manner that allowed determination of the proportion of children whose performance was below normal limits.

The studies just described are limited because they only focus on motor behavior during the first three years of life. The present paper builds on this previous work by exploring whether prenatal opioid exposure is related to poor motor performance during middle childhood. The data will come from longitudinal follow-up of the Chicago sample of infants described above.

METHODS

Sample

The sample consisted of eight- to eleven-year-old African-American children (mean age 120.4 months, SD = 8.9 months, range 107 to 141 months) who had been followed longitudinally since birth. Thirty-five of the children had a documented history of prenatal exposure to opioid drugs; 41 were unexposed to opioids prenatally. All families were recruited into the study between 1978 and 1982 through the obstetrical clinics at Chicago Lying-In Hospital. At the time of recruitment into the study, all families were living in inner-city neighborhoods and were of low to very-low socioeconomic status.

Opioid Group. The opioid-group families were recruited from a special high-risk obstetrical clinic for women abusing drugs. All women who were identified to be using methadone and/or other opioid drugs and who indicated willingness to participate in the research for a period of two years were enrolled in the study. The women were all involved in low-dose methadone-maintenance programs; their dosages during pregnancy ranged from 3 to 40 mg per 24-hour period with a mean of 20 mg. Most of the women using methadone occasionally used other drugs in addition to methadone, most commonly alcohol, marijuana, heroin, cocaine, diazepam, and pentazocine. At the time of birth, the sample contained 36 low-income, African-American, women using methadone who gave birth to 42 infants during the course of the study (including one set of twins). An additional group of three women who delivered four infants were recruited whose primary drug of abuse during pregnancy was the partial opioid-agonist pentazocine (Talwin). In the early 1980s "T's and Blues" (Talwin and an antihistamine)[39] was being widely used on the streets of Chicago as an inexpensive substitute for heroin. For the present report, the children exposed to "T's and Blues" are being included as part of the opioid group because they did not differ noticeably from those exposed to methadone on any of the outcome measures. Five children were lost to the sample within the first six months of life: one died neonatally from a congenital birth defect, one died neonatally from Sudden Infant Death Syndrome (SIDS), two died post-neonatally from SIDS, and one suffered massive brain damage from a stroke at age 4 months. An additional four children were lost to the sample at a later age, mostly through refusals of foster caregivers to allow children to participate in the study. Two children who were participants in the study at age ten did not complete the motor assessments: one whose foster mother did not want her child to be subjected to unnecessary testing, and one who had a pervasive developmental disorder and was unable to follow instructions. Thus motor measures were available at the middle-childhood assessment for thirty-five out of the forty-six children recruited prenatally.

Comparison Group. A comparison group was selected by randomly screening pregnant African-American women attending a clinic at Chicago Lying-In Hospital for low-income, but medically-low-risk obstetrical patients. Women were considered eligible for the comparison group only if they reported never having used opioid drugs, if they were light drinkers or abstainers from alcohol, and if they had no obvious mental retardation or mental illness. Urine screens during pregnancy were used to confirm maternal self-report of drug use. Altogether, 43 women were enrolled in the drug- and alcohol-free comparison group. These women gave birth to 47 infants during the course of the study (including one set of twins). An additional seven women who delivered seven infants met our criteria for the comparison group, although their male partners were either drug or alcohol users. Thirteen children, from the above 54, were lost to follow-up by age ten as a result of problems locating families and refusal of caregivers to allow the children to participate in the study. Thus motor assessments were available at the middle-childhood assessment for forty-one out of the 54 comparison children originally recruited prenatally.

Procedure

At the middle-childhood assessment, children came to a research laboratory located at a community hospital for three two- to three-hour assessment sessions. During the first session, children were administered an intelligence test, followed by a number of quantifiable motor tasks. During the second session children were administered a psychiatric interview. During the third session children were administered a clinical neurological examination, followed by a number of tests of attention. In this paper we will report data from the neurological assessment (the PANESS) and a motor steadiness assessment.

Motor Measures

PANESS. The Revised Physical and Neurological Examination for Soft Signs (PANESS)[40] was administered to all of the children. This instrument was developed by staff at Abbott Laboratories, the National Institute of Mental Health, and the National Institute of Neurological and Communicative Disorders and Stroke in response to a perceived need for a relatively brief, standard assessment of neurological soft signs that could be used across studies. The PANESS includes tasks typical of those used in pediatric examination for minor neurological signs[41] and has been recommended for use in studies of the effects of pharmacologic agents on children's behavior.[40] Data are available on the PANESS from normal populations, but the authors recommend that these be used as guidelines for interpretation rather than as normative standards appropriate for all populations.[40]

In the present study the PANESS was administered by one of the authors (MPG), a physical therapist who was masked to all information about the children's drug exposure or early developmental histories. For purposes of this study, this primary observer established reliability with a secondary observer, a child psychiatrist who had advanced training in child neurology. The two observers first administered PANESS items together to five children, achieving consensus on appropriate administration of items and high agreement (greater than 90%) on scoring of the items involving clinical judgment. Periodically throughout the course of the study, videotapes made of PANESS sessions conducted by the primary observer were rated by the second observer. Again, there were high levels of agreement between the observers.

The PANESS focuses on three domains of motor functioning. The first set of tasks is designed to determine *lateral preference patterns*. Eleven items were administered in which the child was asked to show the examiner how to perform a variety of activities such as combing hair, throwing a ball, and flipping a coin. Based on these items, a child was classified as being right-handed, left-handed, or of mixed laterality (if fewer than seven items were performed with each hand).

The second set of tasks on the PANESS involve assessment of *gross motor coordination, motor overflow, and balance* in a variety of gaits and stations. The gait tasks are a modified Fog Test[42-43] in which children are asked to walk on a line 10 feet long on their heels, on their toes, with feet everted, with feet in tandem going forward, and with feet in tandem going backwards. Two scores were derived from the Fog Test: the number of errors the child made across the tasks (missing the line, not on heels, etc.) and the number of tasks in which the examiner noted associated movements in the arms and hands. Measures of balance were derived from two additional stations tasks. Children were asked to stand for 20 seconds heel-to-foot with eyes closed while the examiner noticed any tendency to fall. The children were asked to stand on each foot for up to 30 seconds while the examiner recorded time before losing balance. The PANESS also includes hopping on one foot tasks, but in the present study these were not coded because of problems in the scoring sheet used.

The third set of tasks on the PANESS includes *timed maneuvers*.[44-45] In these the child was instructed to perform six different timed maneuvers on each side of the body (a total of 12 trials) as fast as possible until told to stop. For each trial, the examiner timed with a stop watch how long it took to accomplish 20 complete movements. Three of the tasks involved repetition of the same action: foot tapping, hand patting, and finger tapping. Three of the tasks involved alternation of movements: heel-toe tap, pronation-supination of hand, and successive finger tapping. In addition to scoring the time to complete twenty of each task on both right and left, the investigator noted for each of the trials whether there were any mirror movements and whether there were lapses in the rhythm of the repetitions or alternations.

Wisconsin Fine Motor Steadiness Battery. Two subtests from the Wisconsin Fine Motor Steadiness Battery were employed in the present study:[46-47] the grooved maze board and the grooved peg board. The battery was designed to assess the movement behavior correlates of brain dysfunction in children, and the motor steadiness tasks have been widely used in the neuropsychological assessment of children.[48] Some normative data on the tasks are available for normal and brain-damaged populations.[49-51] We chose the steadiness tasks for use in this study because they had previously been shown to be sensitive to the effects of children's prenatal exposure to alcohol.[52]

In the *grooved maze board task*, the children were required to move an electronic stylus through a grooved maze with 26 turns and no blind alleys. The groove was 4 mm wide. The maze was on a 23-cm by 28-cm board placed on a stand at a 45 degree angle. An electronic counter, which emitted a beep whenever the stylus touched the side of the groove, recorded the number of errors and time in error for each task. The children were not permitted to rest their arm on the table or support their arm in any way. The task was given twice for each hand. Two scores, number of errors and cumulative time in error, were coded for each hand. Children were told that the purpose of the task was not to see how fast they could complete the maze, but rather how carefully they could complete it without touching the sides.

The *grooved peg board* test required the child to place 25 small, grooved pegs into slots on a 10-cm by 10-cm metal board. All of the pegs had identical grooves, but the corresponding grooves on the holes on the board were rotated in varying positions so that the pegs could only fit in a particular orientation. Children were encouraged to complete the task as quickly as possible. The total time to insert the pegs was recorded for each hand.

RESULTS

Differences Between Opioid-Exposed and Comparison Groups

Our approach to data analysis was to examine differences in mean scores between children who were opioid-exposed and comparison children on each of the dependent motor variables. We also chose to give particular attention to two demographic variables that have a known relationship to neuromotor behavior: sex of child and age of child. If in exploratory analyses either sex or age were related to the motoric variables, we planned to control for them statistically in examining the relationship between prenatal exposure and behavioral outcome.

PANESS. The top portion of Table 2 presents a list of the PANESS summary scores used as dependent variables in data analysis. Right- and left-side trials were summed after preliminary analyses showed no lateralized effects. None of the PANESS variables were significantly correlated with child's sex, although some of the scores were related to age, with older children having faster times. Table 2 provides the point biserial correlations between sex and each of the PANESS items, and correlations between age in months and the PANESS items.

Analyses of covariance (ANCOVAs) were computed on the PANESS subscales using prenatal opioid exposure as a categorical independent variable and age in months as a continuous independent variable after first conducting preliminary analyses confirming that there were no age by drug group interaction effects. In these ANCOVAs there were no significant effects at $p \leq .05$ for prenatal exposure on any of the PANESS variables. There were significant effects for age on time to complete repetitive hand pats ($F(1,73) = 10.76$), time to complete repetitive finger taps ($F(1,73) = 11.85$), dysrhythmia in the repetitive tasks ($F(1,73) = 9.46$), and time to complete successive finger taps ($F(1,73) = 11,35$). The mean PANESS scores by drug-exposure groups are presented in Table 3.

Motor Steadiness. Six motor steadiness variables were subjected to analysis: time in error on the maze, number of errors on the maze, time to complete on the peg board, for both dominant and non-dominant hands. None of the six motor steadiness measures were correlated with sex. Significant correlations between the age of the child in months and the four maze measures were found. These are reported in Table 2.

Before computing ANCOVAs on the motor steadiness measures, preliminary analyses were used to determine whether there were any age by drug exposure group interactions. For one of the dependent variables, dominant hand time on peg board, there was a significant age by exposure interaction effect ($F(1,72) = 7.4$, $p \leq .05$). Because of this interaction effect, the sample was dichotomized near the median for age in months:

TABLE 2. Sex and Age Correlations with Motor Scores

Scale	Sex[#]	Age
PANESS Gaits and Stations		
Errors across 5 gait tasks	0.07	−0.13
Number of gait tasks showing overflow	0.09	0.13
Tendency to fall in standing heel-to-toe	0.03	0.15
Unable to balance on either foot for 20 seconds	0.06	−0.17
Unable to balance on either foot for 10 seconds	0.20	−0.14
PANESS Timed Movements		
Foot tap: time for 20 right and left	−0.04	−0.22*
Hand pat time for 20 right and left	0.24*	−0.36*
Finger tap: time for 20 right and left	0.12	−0.38**
Number of repetitive trials showing dysrhythmia	0.15	−0.36**
Number of repetitive trials showing motor overflow	−0.01	−0.16
Foot-heel-toe tap: time for 20 right and left	0.10	−0.15
Hand pronation/supination: time for 20 right and left	−0.01	−0.19
Finger succession: time for 20 right and left	−0.12	−0.38**
Number of alternating trials showing dysrhythmia	0.13	−0.11
Number of alternating trials showing motor overflow	0.07	−0.14
Motor Steadiness Summary Scores		
Maze Time in Error: dominant hand	0.03	−0.46**
Maze Time in Error: non-dominant hand	0.14	−0.34*
Maze Number of Errors: dominant hand	0.09	−0.49**
Maze Number of Errors: non-dominant hand	0.14	−0.34*
Peg Board Time to Complete: dominant hand	0.05	−0.24*
Peg Board Time to Complete: non-dominant hand	0.14	−0.14

* $p \leq .05$
** $p \leq .01$
# Sex was coded so that 1 = male and 2 = female

younger children were those between 107 and 120 months, older children were those between 121 and 141 months.

F tests were computed examining drug exposure effects for each of the six dependent variables separately for older and younger children. No significant exposure effects were found for the older children. There were, however, significant prenatal exposure effects for the younger children on the dominant hand time on maze ($F(1,34) = 4.6$, $p \leq .05$); dominant hand errors on maze ($F(1,34) = 4.0$, $p \leq .05$); dominant hand time on peg board

TABLE 3. PANESS Scale Scores by Prenatal Opioid Exposure

PANESS Subscale	Opioid Group		Comparison Group	
Manual Lateral Preference	Frequencies			
Right	31		37	
Left	3		2	
Mixed	1		2	
Gaits and Stations Tasks	Means and (Standard Deviations)			
Errors across 5 gait tasks	3.02	(2.85)	3.37	(3.00)
Number of gait tasks showing overflow	3.03	(1.74)	2.80	(1.52)
	Frequencies and Percentages			
Unable to balance on either foot for 20 seconds	28	(80.0%)	32	(78.1%)
Unable to balance on either foot for 10 seconds	17	(48.6%)	18	(43.9%)
Tendency to fall in standing heel-to-toe task	10	(28.6%)	14	(34.2%)
Timed Repetitive Maneuvers	Means and (Standard Deviations)			
Foot Tap: time for 20 right and left	12.17	(2.69)	12.14	(3.36)
Hand Pat: time for 20 right and left	9.49	(1.66)	9.03	(1.80)
Finger Tap: time for 20 right and left	12.71	(2.04)	11.98	(1.81)
Number of trials showing dysrhythmia	1.41	(1.16)	1.03	(1.16)
Number of trials showing motor overflow	1.21	(1.34)	1.36	(1.39)
Timed Alternating Maneuvers	Means and (Standard Deviations)			
Foot-heel-toe tap: time for 20 right and left	15.44	(4.14)	14.58	(4.20)
Hand pronation/supination: time 20 right and left	12.78	(1.89)	12.48	(2.90)
Finger succession	17.88	(3.91)	17.65	(4.88)
Number of trials showing dysrhythmia	3.59	(1.34)	3.46	(1.50)
Number of trials showing motor overflow	1.94	(1.60)	1.33	(1.26)

$(F(1,34) = 7.42, p \leq .05)$; and non-dominant hand time on peg board $(F(1,34) = 4.2, p \leq .05)$. On each of these assessments the younger children who were prenatally exposed performed more poorly than the younger comparison children. Table 4 includes the mean performance on the motor steadiness tasks for the drug groups by age.

Finally, in order to explore further the possible mechanism by which prenatal exposure might lead to performance deficits on the motor steadiness tasks, we examined whether these deficits in the younger children might be

TABLE 4. Motor Steadiness Summary Scores by Prenatal Opioid Exposure

Measure	Hand	Younger Opioid Mean & (SD)	Younger Comparison Mean & (SD)	Older Opioid Mean & (SD)	Older Comparison Mean & (SD)
		n = 15	n = 21	n = 20	n = 20
Maze Time in Error	Dominant Hand	6.08* (3.32)	3.86 (2.84)	3.16 (2.54)	3.27 (2.89)
	Non-Dominant Hand	9.09 (3.17)	7.77 (5.21)	7.11 (5.13)	7.40 (4.98)
Maze Number of Errors	Dominant Hand	32.07* (14.91)	22.38 (13.97)	18.68 (13.30)	15.39 (12.45)
	Non-Dominant Hand	49.80 (16.18)	42.67 (23.00)	44.05 (33.89)	36.06 (17.35)
Peg Board Time to Complete	Dominant Hand	103.8* (20.69)	88.38 (13.3)	87.4 (16.12)	92.56 (17.97)
	Non-Dominant Hand	110.20* (16.75)	98.46 (17.18)	98.10 (19.34)	102.58 (22.64)

* Younger children who were opioid-exposed performed significantly more poorly than younger comparison children on these tasks

mediated by lower birth weight. The opioid-exposed group had been significantly smaller at birth than the comparison group [opioid mean: 2867 g (SD = 596); comparison mean: 3197 g (SD = 338), t = 3.01, p ≤ .01]. ANCOVAs were computed on the six motor steadiness measures using exposure history as the categorical independent variable and entering birth weight as a continuous covariate. After controlling for birth weight, exposure remained significantly or marginally significantly related to the three motor steadiness measures on the dominant hand measures (time on maze ($F(1,32) = 3.7$, $p \leq .06$); errors on maze ($F(1,32) = 3.4$, $p \leq .07$); and time on peg board ($F(1,32) = 4.4$, $p \leq .05$)), but not to the non-dominant hand measures.

Clinical Profile of Methadone-Exposed Children with Poor Motor Functioning

The analyses presented above were computed in order to explore the hypothesis that prenatal methadone exposure has a long-term effect on the motor behavior of children. Analyses of this sort have two deficiencies: (1) by relying on reports of means, they obscure variability within groups, and (2) they provide no anchor points for determining the clinical significance of the findings. Because the instruments used in this study were not formally normed or referenced to particular clinical populations, the children in this study cannot be directly compared with any known population of children.

The following three case vignettes are presented in an effort to describe the range of functioning between the best and worst functioning children in the methadone-exposed group and also to describe the clinical heterogeneity of the children with the poorer levels of functioning. Two boys (Darius and Marcus) are described whose scores on the motor steadiness tasks placed them in the bottom fifth of the sample, and one boy (Danny) whose scores placed him in the top fifth of the sample.

Darius was born prematurely weighing only 1280 grams, making him the smallest child at birth in the research sample. He showed clear signs of narcotics withdrawal neonatally and during the first two years of life lagged in his acquisition of motor milestones, with Bayley PDI scores ranging from 75 to 88. At age ten Darius showed poor balance on the PANESS, a high degree of overflow on the Fog Test and timed maneuvers, and very poor scores on the motor steadiness tasks. His intellectual performance, however, was normal as measured by the Wechsler Intelligence Scales for Children-Revised (WISC-R):[53] 101 verbal IQ and 90 performance IQ. On a computerized vigilance test, the Continuous Performance Test,[54] his performance was in the normal range. His teachers noticed occasional disruptive behavior in the classroom, but generally found him to be a child who "puts pride in his work and enjoys being recognized as a good student." Although his mother noted that he was not particularly athletic and avoided participating in sports, his motor impairments were in no way a serious handicap to him at school or with his peers.

Marcus was born at term weighing 2750 grams. His delivery had been complicated by breech position and abnormal heart tones, and his Apgar scores were 6 at one minute and 8 at five minutes. Throughout the first month of life he showed clear signs of narcotics withdrawal. Marcus achieved all of his motor milestones on time during infancy, achieving Bayley PDI scores consistently higher than 90. At age ten Marcus had difficulty with portions of the PANESS. Although he wrote with his left hand, Marcus indicated that he would perform seven out of the eleven manual tasks with his right hand. He demonstrated clear motor overflow on the gait tasks and during timed maneuvers. He was unable to stand still for the test of static balance. His scores were very poor on the motor steadiness tasks. Marcus's general level of intellectual functioning was borderline; he had a verbal IQ of 82 and performance IQ of 64. His performance was especially poor on the digit span, arithmetic, and coding subscales—tests that require the ability to maintain good attention and concentration for successful completion. On a computerized vigilance task, Marcus made many impulsive errors. Although he was affable and polite to the examiners, he seemed quite emotionally labile and had a great deal of trouble staying on task. Examiners commented that he squirmed and moved throughout the testing sessions. His problems with inhibitory control seemed to cross cognitive, fine motor, gross motor, and emotional domains. In school he was placed in a classroom for children with emotional disturbance.

Danny was born at term after an uncomplicated pregnancy weighing 2750 grams. He showed clear signs of neonatal withdrawal. During the first two years of life he achieved his motor milestones on time, with PDI scores consistently above 90. At age 11 Danny performed quite well on the motor steadiness tasks and the PANESS except that he had trouble standing on one foot and standing heel-toe with eyes closed. His scores on the timed maneuvers and computerized vigilance tests were excellent. His verbal IQ was 94 and performance 93. At school Danny was performing below grade level and was of great concern to his teachers because of his disruptive behavior.

DISCUSSION

We began this study with the hypothesis that children prenatally exposed to opioids would show deficits in motor behavior during middle childhood. Previous studies of infants exposed prenatally to opioids have repeatedly demonstrated the dramatic effects of the drug on motoric behavior in the first days and weeks after birth.[14-24] Several studies have also suggested that infants who were opioid-exposed might have delays in motor development and the presence of neurological soft signs during the first two years after birth,[30-35] although findings have varied across studies and generally point to larger opioid effects during the second year of life. The data presented in this paper provide partial support for the hypothesis that prenatal exposure to opioids is related to motor deficits at school age. With the measures we employed, methadone exposure effects were clearly observable in the younger children in the sample, but not in those who had passed their tenth birthdays.

Why were opioid exposure effects only observable in the younger children in the present sample? Middle childhood is a period of many changes in performance on neuromotor tasks[41,44-45,55-56] and a time of documented psychobiological changes, such as those in corpus callosum functioning,[57] that might affect performance on complex tasks. We suspect that developmental shifts in neuromotor competence occur during middle childhood that are related to performance on the maze and peg board tasks used in this study. Specifically, if methadone exposure causes not a permanent deficit in ability to perform such complex tasks, but rather a delay in acquisition of ability, one would expect a pattern of results similar to what we found. Developmental data on the motor steadiness tests reported by Knights and Moule[50] suggest rapid age-related improvement in performance from ages five to nine, at which time performance plateaus to mature levels. The data in the present study suggest that opioid-exposed children might reach their level of mature performance on this test by age ten rather than age nine, as comparison children did.

The data presented in this study provide little information on the specific types of underlying competencies that are lacking or delayed in younger children who were opioid-exposed. The name of the motor steadiness battery clearly implies that hand steadiness is crucial to performance of the tasks, but other abilities are demanded by these tasks as well. The maze and pegboard tasks require considerable visual-spatial perceptual skills as well as the capacity to integrate visual-spatial information with motoric responses. The error-corrective component of the tasks, particularly the maze tasks, is also important. Correction of errors requires the rapid inhibition of movement followed by controlled activation of antagonistic muscle groups. This type of control process has been described in other work using the peg board tasks[58] as well as work on tapping[59] and aiming at a target.[60]

The present study suggests that at least some motoric measures may be sensitive markers of teratologic effects on central nervous system development after infancy. One other long-term follow-up study of substance-exposed children also confirms the sensitivity of motoric measures to teratologic effects. In the Seattle Longitudinal Study on Alcohol and Pregnancy[52] 457 four-year-old children were administered a battery of motor tests that included the Wisconsin Motor Steadiness Battery. Children were also administered a battery of gross motor tasks, not unlike those on the PANESS. At age four, after controlling for other confounding variables, moderate levels of prenatal alcohol exposure were related to increased errors and increased total time on the Wisconsin Fine Motor Steadiness Battery and poorer balance but not coordination on the Gross Motor Scale.

The results of the Seattle alcohol study and the Chicago opioid study suggest that the types of motor functions assessed by neurological tests such as the PANESS, in particular gross motor coordination and motor overflow, may be relatively invulnerable to the effects of prenatal drug and alcohol exposure. Alternatively, the insensitivity of the PANESS and the relatively greater sensitivity of the Wisconsin Motor Steadiness battery may be related to issues other than the types of functions the instruments tap. Perhaps the greater sensitivity of the motor steadiness tasks may result from the capacity of the tests to detect deviations not easily observed by the human eye or to the more challenging nature, and hence greater age-appropriateness, of the tasks on the steadiness battery. Just as the measures of steadiness were not sensitive to prenatal exposure effects after the age of ten, simpler tasks on the PANESS might have been sensitive indicators of prenatal exposure with children younger than the nine- and ten-year-olds we studied. More complex gross motor and balance tasks might have been appropriate for the older children in our sample. Our data illustrate the importance in behavioral teratology studies of carefully matching the instrument to the age expectations of the child.

Finally, although the data presented in this paper demonstrate that pre-natal exposure to opioids may have long-term motor consequences, the clinical application of these findings is not immediately obvious. What is the impact of these deficits on the lives of the affected children? How should practitioners intervene with children who were prenatally drug-exposed when they are encountered at different stages in the life cycle?

The statistical analyses and case vignettes presented in this paper suggest that children born to users of heroin and methadone do not suffer profound disturbances in the motoric domain except during the neonatal period. By middle childhood, the types of behavioral signs observed in the children in this sample were not unique to drug-exposed children, but rather of the same sort that are commonly seen in special education and clinical settings. The techniques that might be used with such children are the same as those already used by practitioners to deal with children who have minor motor deficits, attention deficit disorder, or special educational problems.

By middle childhood, children with prenatal drug exposure differ great-ly from one another in their patterns of neurobehavioral functioning. There is no prototypic drug-exposed child. Many children show little or no impairment whatsoever. Two of the children presented in the case vi-gnettes had clear motoric deficits, but were quite different from one anoth-er. These children, both performing extremely poorly on the motor steadi-ness tasks, had greatly differing developmental histories, patterns of soft neurological signs during middle childhood, and functional outcomes. One child's impairment was limited to the motoric domain; the other child's problems extended more broadly to a cluster of deficits related to inhibitory control. The differences between the two children illustrate the importance of looking beyond a single domain in assessing the effects of drug exposure, of focusing on problems of true functional significance, and of approaching each child as a unique case in designing an intervention. Because of the great heterogeneity of developmental histories and outcomes in children with prenatal drug exposure, it is difficult to outline a standard set of intervention techniques. Interventions need to be tailored to a particular child and family to help that child to better organize behavior and hence increase his or her ability to be effectively involved with the environment and to experience a sense of competence.

ACKNOWLEDGMENTS

The authors gratefully acknowledge the role played by Joseph Marcus, MD, in initiating this longitudinal study and in providing us with major support and guidance in conducting the neurological assessment at the middle-childhood follow-up. We also acknowledge the role of Linda Henson and Karen Freel in coordinating the assessment of families throughout the many years of this project.

This research was funded through NIDA grant R01 DA05396 to Sydney Hans. Mary Grattan's work on this project was in part supported by a fellowship from the National Center for Clinical Infant Programs, Zero to Three.

REFERENCES

1. Zuckerman B, Frank D. "Crack kids": Not broken. *Pediatr.* 1992;89:337-339.

2. Vorhees CV. Origins of behavioral teratology. In: Riley EP, Vorhees CV eds. *Handbook of Behavioral Teratology.* New York, NY: Plenum Press; 1986;3-22.

3. Adams J. Methods in behavioral teratology. In: Riley EP, Vorhees CV eds. *Handbook of Behavioral Teratology.* New York, NY: Plenum Press; 1986;67-97.

4. Jacobson JL, Jacobson SW. Methodological issues in human behavioral teratology. In: Rovee-Collier C, Lipsitt LP eds. *Advances in Infancy Research,* vol. 6. Norwood, NJ: Ablex; 1990;111-148.

5. Hertzig ME. Neurological 'soft' signs in low birth-weight children. *Dev Med Child Neurol.* 1981;23:778-791.

6. Marlow N, Roberts L, Cooke R. Outcome at 8 years for children with birth weights of 1250 or less. *Arch Dis Child.* 1993;68:286-289.

7. Zagon IS, McLaughlin PJ. An overview of the neurobehavioral sequelae of perinatal opioid exposure. In: Yanai J ed. *Neurobehavioral Teratology.* Amsterdam: Elsevier; 1984:197-233.

8. Martin M, Hecker J, Clark R. China white epidemic: An eastern United States emergency department experience. *Ann Emergency Med.* 1991;20:158-164.

9. Hutchings DE. *Methadone: A Treatment for Drug Addiction.* New York, NY: Chelsea House; 1985.

10. Blinick G, Inturrisi CE, Jerez E, Wallach RC. Methadone assays in pregnant women and progeny. *Am J Obstet Gynecol.* 1975;121:617-621.

11. Desmond MM, Wilson GS. Neonatal abstinence syndrome: Recognition and diagnosis. *Addict Dis.* 1975;2:113-121.

12. Finnegan LP, Kron RE, Connaughton JF, Jr, Emich JP. Neonatal abstinence syndrome: Assessment and management. In: Harbison RD ed. *Perinatal Addiction.* New York, NY: Spectrum Publications; 1975; 141-158.

13. Brazelton TB. Neonatal Behavioral Assessment Scale, 2nd ed. Philadelphia, PA: Lippincott, 1984.

14. Soule AB III, Standley K, Copans SA, Davis M. Clinical uses of the Brazelton Neonatal Scale. *Pediatr.* 1974;54:583-586.

15. Strauss ME, Lessen-Firestone JK, Starr RH, Ostrea EM, Jr. Behavior of narcotics addicted newborns. *Child Dev.* 1975;46:887-893.

16. Strauss ME, Starr RH, Ostrea EM, Jr, Chavez CJ, Stryker JC. Behavioral concomitants of prenatal addiction to narcotics. *J Pediatr.* 1976;89:842-846.

17. Kron RE, Kaplan SL, Finnegan LP, Litt M, Phoenix MD. The assessment of behavioral change in infants undergoing narcotic withdrawal: Comparative data from clinical and objective methods. *Addict Dis.* 1975;2:257-275.

18. Kron RE, Kaplan SL, Phoenix MD, Finnegan LP. Behavior of infants born to drug-dependent mothers: Effects of prenatal and postnatal drugs. In: Rementeria JL ed. *Drug Abuse in Pregnancy and Neonatal Effects.* St. Louis, MO: Moseley; 1977:129-144.

19. Chasnoff IJ, Hatcher R, Burns WJ. Early growth patterns of methadone-addicted infants. *Am J Dis Child,* 1980;134:1049-1051.

20. Chasnoff IJ, Hatcher R, Burns WJ. Polydrug- and methadone-addicted newborns: A continuum of impairment? *Pediatr.* 1982;70:210-213.

21. Jeremy RJ, Hans SL. Behavior of neonates exposed in utero to methadone as assessed on the Brazelton scale. *Inf Behav Dev.* 1985;8:323-336.

22. Lesser-Katz M. Some effects of maternal drug addiction on the neonate. *Int J Addict.* 1982;17:887-896.

23. Lodge A, Marcus MM, Ramer CM. Behavioral and electrophysiological characteristics of the addicted neonate. *Addict Dis.* 1975;2:235-255.

24. Marcus J, Hans, SL. Electromyographic assessment of neonatal muscle tone. *Psychiatr Res.* 1982;6:31-40.

25. Zagon IS, McLaughlin PJ. Perinatal methadone exposure and its influence on the behavioral ontogeny of rats. *Pharmacol Biochem Behavior.* 1978;9:665-672.

26. Walz MA, Davis WM, Pace HB. Prenatal methadone treatment: a multigenerational study of development and behavior in offspring. *Dev Pharmacol Ther.* 1983;6:125-137.

27. Handelmann GE, Dow-Edwards D. Modulation of brain development by morphine: Effects on central motor system and behavior. *Peptides.* 1985;Suppl:29-34.

28. Newby-Schmidt MB, Norton S. Alterations of chick locomotion produced by morphine treatment in ovo. *Neurotoxicology.* 1981;2:743-748.

29. Bayley N. *Manual for the Bayley Scales of Infant Development.* New York, NY: Psychological Corporation; 1969.

30. Strauss ME, Starr RH, Ostrea EM, Jr, Chavez CJ, Stryker JC. Behavioral concomitants of prenatal addiction to narcotics. *J Pediatr.* 1976;89:842-846.

31. Wilson GS, Desmond MM, Wait RB. Follow-up of methadone-treated and untreated narcotic-dependent women and their infants: Health, developmental, and social implications. *J Pediatr.* 1981;98:716-722.

32. Rosen TS, Johnson HL. Children of methadone-maintained mothers: Follow-up to 18 months of age. *J Pediatr.* 1982;101:192-196.

33. Johnson HL, Diano A, Rosen TS. 24-month neurobehavioral follow-up of children of methadone-maintained mothers. *Inf Behav Dev.* 1984;7:115-123.

34. Johnson HL, Glassman MB, Fiks KB, Rosen T. Path analysis of variables affecting 36-month outcome in a population of multi-risk children. *Inf Behav Dev.* 1987;10:451-465.

35. Hans SL. Maternal opioid drug use and child development. In: Zagon IS, Slotkin TA eds. *Maternal Substance Abuse and the Developing Nervous System.* New York, NY: Academic Press; 1992:177-213.

36. Marcus J, Hans SL, Jeremy RJ. A longitudinal study of offspring born to methadone-maintained women: III. Effects of multiple risk factors on development at four, eight, and twelve months. *Am J Alcohol Drug Abuse.* 1984;10:195-207.

37. Marcus J, Hans SL, Jeremy RJ. Patterns of 1-day and 4-month motor functioning in infants of women on methadone. *Neurobehavioral Toxicology and Teratology.* 1982;4:473-476.

38. Hans SL. Developmental consequences of prenatal exposure to methadone. *Ann NY Acad Sci.* 1989;562:195-207.

39. Chasnoff IF, Hatcher R, Burns WJ, Schnoll SH. Pentazocine and tripellannamine ("T's and Blues"): Effects on the fetus and neonate. *Dev Pharm Therapeutics.* 1983;6:162-169.

40. Denckla MB. Revised neurological examination for subtle signs. *Psychopharmacology Bull.* 1985;21:773-792.

41. Wolff PH, Gunnoe C, Cohen C. Neuromotor maturation and psychological performance: A developmental study. *Dev Med Child Neurol.* 1985;27:344-354.

42. Fog E, Fog M. Cerebral inhibition examined by associated movements. In: Bax M, MacKeith R eds. *Minimal Cerebral Dysfunction. Clinics in Developmental Medicine No. 10.* London: S.I.M.P. with Heinemann Medical; 1963.

43. Szatmari P, Taylor DC. Overflow movements and behavior problems: Scoring and using a modification of Fogs' Test. *Dev Med Child Neurol.* 1984;26:297-310.

44. Denckla MB. Development of speed in repetitive and successive finger-movements in normal children. *Dev Med Child Neurol.* 1973;15:635-645.

45. Denckla MB. Development of motor co-ordination in normal children. *Dev Med Child Neurol.* 1974;16:729-741.

46. Matthews CG, Cleeland CS, Hopper CL. Neuropsychological patterns in multiple sclerosis. *Diseases of the Nervous System.* 1970;31:161-170.

47. Matthews CG, Klove H. *Wisconsin Motor Steadiness Battery. Administration Manual for Child Neuropsychology Battery.* Madison, WI: University of Wisconsin Medical School, Neuropsychology Laboratory; 1978.

48. Klove H. Clinical neuropsychology. In: Forster FM ed. *The Medical Clinics of North America.* New York, NY: Saunders; 1963:1647-1658.

49. Gaddes WH. Normative data on a number of psychological tests. Victoria, British Columbia: University of Victoria Neuropsychological Laboratory; 1966.

50. Knights RM, Moule AD. Normative data on the motor steadiness battery for children. *Perceptual Motor Skills.* 1968;26:643-650.

51. Trites RL, Price MA. *Assessment of Readiness for Primary French Immersion.* Ottawa, Canada: University of Ottawa Press; 1978.

52. Barr HM, Streissguth AP, Darby BL, Sampson PD. Prenatal exposure to alcohol, caffeine, tobacco, and aspirin: Effects on fine and gross motor performance in 4-year-old children. *Dev Psychol.* 1990;26:339-348.

53. Wechsler D. *Manual for the Wechsler Intelligence Scale for Children-Revised.* New York, NY: Psychological Corporation; 1974.

54. Nuechterlein, KH. Signal detection in vigilance tasks and behavioral attributes among offspring of schizophrenic mothers and among hyperactive children. *J Abnormal Psychol.* 1983;92:4-28.

55. Touwen BCL. *Examination of the Child with Minor Neurological Dysfunction.* London: William Heinemann Limited; 1979.

56. Peters JE, Roming JS, Dykman RA. A special neurological examination of children with learning disabilities. *Dev Med Child Neurol.* 1974;175:63-75.

57. Kohn B, Dennis M. Selective impairments of visuo-spatial abilities in infantile hemiplegics after right cerebral hemidecortication. *Neuropsychologia.* 1974;12:505-512.

58. Annett J, Annett, Hudson P, Turner A. The control of movement in the preferred and non-preferred hands. *Quarterly J Exp Psychol.* 1979;31:641-651.

59. Peters M. Why the preferred hand taps more quickly than the non-preferred hand: three experiments on handedness. *Canadian J Psychol.* 1980;34:62-71.

60. Todor J, Cisneros J. Accommodation to increased accuracy demands by the right and left hands. *J Motor Behavior.* 1985;17:355-372.

Adolescent Pregnancy
and the Complications
of Prenatal Substance Use

Marie D. Cornelius

SUMMARY. Pregnancy in a teenager presents increased risks for both mother and offspring. When a pregnant teenager also uses drugs, tobacco, alcohol or a combination of these substances, results are especially problematic. This paper reviews the complications of adolescent pregnancy, rates of teenage use of commonly abused substances, and data on effects of prenatal substance abuse in adolescents on gestational length and on growth and development of offspring. *[Article copies available from The Haworth Document Delivery Service: 1-800-342-9678. E-mail address: getinfo@haworth.com]*

Teenage pregnancy is prevalent and increasing. The rate of births to adolescents in 1991 rose for the fifth consecutive year, to 62 births per 1000 teenagers.[1] Data from the Centers for Disease Control, Youth Risk Behavior Survey[2] indicated that 52% of the females reported first sexual intercourse before age 17 which may presage future increases in teenage pregnancy. In addition, drug and alcohol use is quite common among adolescents. Seventy-seven percent of high school seniors in the United States drank alcohol, 28% smoked tobacco, and 22% used marijuana in 1992.[3] The combination of the prevalences of teenage pregnancy and

Marie D. Cornelius, PhD, is Assistant Professor, Departments of Psychiatry and Epidemiology, Western Psychiatric Institute and Clinic, Program in Epidemiology, Pittsburgh, PA 15213.

[Haworth co-indexing entry note]: "Adolescent Pregnancy and the Complications of Prenatal Substance Abuse." Cornelius, Marie D. Co-published simultaneously in *Physical & Occupational Therapy in Pediatrics* (The Haworth Press, Inc.) Vol. 16, No. 1/2, 1996, pp. 111-128; and: *Children with Prenatal Drug Exposure* (ed: Lynette S. Chandler, and Shelly J. Lane) The Haworth Press, Inc., 1996, pp. 111-128. Single or multiple copies of this article are available from The Haworth Document Delivery Service [1-800-342-9678, 9:00 a.m. - 5:00 p.m. (EST). E-mail address: getinfo@haworth.com].

© 1996 by The Haworth Press, Inc. All rights reserved.   *111*

adolescent substance use, and the increased risks associated with teenage pregnancy, have ominous implications for the health of the offspring of teen mothers. This paper will: (1) review the complications of adolescent pregnancy in both the offspring and mother; (2) review the adverse effects of prenatal exposure to the most commonly used substances (alcohol, tobacco, marijuana); and (3) report on recent data about adolescent prenatal substance use and effects on their offspring.

ADOLESCENT PREGNANCY AND PARENTHOOD

Effects of Adolescent Pregnancy and Parenthood on the Offspring

Infants of adolescents are two to six times more likely to be low birth weight (LBW) compared to infants of adults. By the time they reach school age, they are also more likely to be below the third percentile for height and weight.[4] During the first year of life, the mortality rate of children born to adolescent mothers is two to three times that of children of older mothers.[5] These children experience an increased incidence of infection, accidental death and violence, and an incidence of sudden infant death syndrome (SIDS) six times greater than that of children born to older mothers.[6]

Consistent evidence shows that children of adolescent mothers are more likely to show cognitive deficits such as lower intellectual ability and school failure, compared with children of older mothers.[7,8] These differences have been shown to worsen as the child ages.[9] By elementary school, children of adolescents are more often described as easily distracted, disorganized, low in frustration tolerance and impulsive, characteristics often associated with being "unready to learn."[10] This finding is of particular importance because retention in grade has been shown to be a critical predictor of later educational and economic success.[9]

Relatively few studies have examined the effect of adolescent pregnancy and parenting on the social and emotional development of children born to adolescent mothers.[11] Data suggest, however, that the children of adolescent mothers are less securely attached and are more often rated by their mothers as having "difficult temperaments" compared with children of older mothers.[12] These findings are important because data derived from research with adult mothers indicate that these indices of early social-emotional development are predictive of later cognitive, educational and social competencies.[13]

Biological risk factors may directly contribute to a risk differential between offspring of teenaged mothers and offspring of mature mothers. The young adolescent is still in a growth spurt which may interfere with shifting necessary nutrition to the fetus.[14,15] In addition, a series of "indirect effects" of young maternal age have been shown to explain a large portion of the variance in outcomes between children of adolescents and those of adult mothers.[16] The "indirect effects" of adolescent parenthood most commonly identified include the lack of access and/or ability to utilize existing health care resources, high environmental stress, low social support, negative parenting attitudes, lack of knowledge about child development, poor parenting skills, relatively poor coping skills, and psychological immaturity.[7]

Effects of Adolescent Childbearing on the Mother

Adolescent mothers are at an increased risk for obstetric complications including toxemia, hypertension, anemia, uterine dysfunction, prolonged labor, urinary tract infections, cephalo-pelvic disproportion, nutritional deficiencies, and use of forceps and Cesarean-section deliveries.[17] Adolescent pregnancy may also result in height retardation in the mother because pregnancy may cause premature epiphyseal closure.[18] Overall, factors such as better socioeconomic status, maternal education and availability of prenatal care and nutrition ameliorate the influence of young maternal age on these outcomes.[19] This protective effect does not, however, hold true for the youngest (i.e., less than 15 years of age) most "at-risk" group of adolescent parents.[7]

The environment of the adolescent mother is characterized by high levels of stress and low levels of personal, familial and societal support.[20] Thus, adolescent mothers must cope with the normative age-related changes of adolescence and the demands of parenthood without the benefit of those supports known to foster adequate coping skills.[21] Compared to peers who delayed childbearing, adolescent mothers are more likely to rely on coping skills which are more passive and avoidant in nature, such as alcohol and drug use.[22,23] In a recent sample of 130 adolescent mothers, the use of drugs was the single most frequent coping mechanism used for managing stress.[24] The use of substances as a coping mechanism is problematic not only because of the immediate effect of the substance, but also because substance use limits the adolescent's ability to mature and to parent.

The use of substances as a coping mechanism prenatally has clear implications for prenatal development and pregnancy outcomes. The effects of continued substance use on the adolescent's experience of parenthood or her child's development is not yet clear, but research does exist which suggests that, for adolescents who have a prior history of relying on drugs as a coping mechanism, the stresses associated with early pregnancy and parenthood may be cause for particular concern.[25] For example, Kaplan and associates[26] found that adolescent mothers who were depressed were at greater risk for substance abuse both during and after pregnancy. These data are of particular relevance given Colletta's findings[27] that 59% of a sample of 75 mothers between the ages of 15 and 19 reported symptoms of depression. Other researchers, such as Zuckerman and colleagues[25] speculate that drug and alcohol use increase in the postpartum period among adolescent mothers.

Substance use and adolescent pregnancy have similar correlates and both are associated with higher rates of school difficulties; conflict in the home; depression; early use of cigarettes, alcohol and drugs; low religiosity; early sexual intercourse; and low parental and high peer influence.[28-30] Because the number of teenage mothers is rising, the absolute number of teen mothers who use substances during pregnancy is also rising. Unfortunately, the preponderance of research on the effects of prenatal exposure to tobacco, alcohol and marijuana have come from studies of adult women. It is, therefore, important to study the actual patterns of substance use among pregnant teenagers and to examine the potential detriment to the offspring.

PRENATAL TOBACCO, ALCOHOL AND MARIJUANA EFFECTS ON THE OFFSPRING

Effects of Prenatal Tobacco on the Offspring

Maternal tobacco use during pregnancy has been associated with growth retardation in the offspring.[31,32] Birthweight decreases in direct proportion to the number of cigarettes smoked.[33] The longer-term effects of prenatal tobacco exposure on the offspring are not as clear. Naeye, analyzing data from the Collaborative Perinatal Project, detected a very small difference in height and head circumference in exposed offspring at age 7.[14] Rantakallio found that exposed offspring were shorter at age 14,[34] and Fogelman and Manor reported decreased height at ages 7, 11, and 23.[35] Others have found no long-term growth retardation.[36,37] In an adult longitudinal study, there was a significant inverse relationship between tobacco use and weight, length, and head circumference at birth.[32] At 8 months of age, only length continued to be associated with prenatal tobacco exposure. By 18 months of age, there was no relationship between prenatal tobacco exposure and size of the offspring.

Findings regarding tobacco exposure and congenital malformations have not been consistent. Based on the outcome of nearly 13,000 pregnancies, Himmelberger and associates reported that the risk of congenital abnormalities increased with increasing levels of maternal smoking.[38] In a large retrospective study of over 288,000 live singleton births, smoking during pregnancy did not increase the odds of congenital malformations.[39]

Kristjansson and colleagues found that prenatal tobacco exposure predicted impulsivity and increased overall activity after controlling for other prenatal drug use and postnatal second-hand smoke.[40] Poor mental scores, poor language development and lower cognitive scores in 2-,[41] 3-, and 4-year-olds[42] were reported for offspring who were prenatally exposed to tobacco. In the cohort of Day and associates,[43,44] prenatal tobacco exposure predicted increased levels of activity, as well as increased oppositional behavior, emotional instability and physical aggression in three-year-olds (unpublished data). In addition, prenatal tobacco exposure significantly predicted increased activity level, inattention, impulsivity and difficult peer relationships among the three-year-old offspring.

Effects of Prenatal Alcohol on the Offspring

Alcohol has been established as a teratogenic agent for the human fetus.[45,46] Prenatal alcohol exposure has been shown to cause morphological, growth, and neurobehavioral abnormalities at birth. In a longitudinal study,[43] prenatal alcohol exposure was significantly related to reduced head circumference and an increased rate of LBW.

Long-term effects of prenatal alcohol exposure in offspring of adult mothers have been reported. Children diagnosed at birth as having fetal alcohol syndrome (FAS) have slower rates of postnatal growth, developmental deficits, and increased rates of minor physical anomalies.[47,48] As they get older, these children continue to have small stature, mental retardation and behavioral problems.[49-51] In the study of Day and colleagues, children who were exposed prenatally to alcohol were smaller at eight months,[52] eighteen months,[53] and thirty-six months of age.[54] Prenatal alcohol exposure has also been associated with motor and intellectual delays and with attention deficits.[51] It has been associated with increased rates of hyperactivity and impulsivity in a sample of five-year-olds.[55] In addition, Coles and associates[56] found that drinking throughout pregnancy affected short-term memory in offspring. In Day and associates' sample of three-year-old offspring of adults, second and third trimester alcohol use predicted a decrease of 8 points on the short-term memory subtest of the Stanford-Binet (Day and associates, unpublished data).

Effects of Prenatal Marijuana on the Offspring

A number of studies have investigated the relationship between prenatal marijuana exposure and birth outcome, but the results of these studies are not consistent.[57] Gestational age has been reported to be shortened by about one week among mothers who use 5+ joints per week as compared to non-using mothers.[58] Another study reported no association between prenatal marijuana use and gestational age, but a slightly elevated risk of pre-term delivery among Caucasian women who were regular users (2+ times per month).[59] In the adult cohort study, no relationship was found between prenatal marijuana use and gestational age;[44] these findings were corroborated by several other researchers.[60-63]

A negative relationship between prenatal marijuana use and neonatal birth weight and length was found by Zuckerman and associates.[64] Hatch and Bracken[59] found a significant risk of LBW among Caucasian offspring. There was no effect, however, on birth weight or head circumference after socioeconomic status, race, other drug use, and maternal age were controlled for in the analysis,[44] although this and another study[60] found a slight negative effect on birth length. No significant effect of prenatal marijuana use on neonatal growth was found in the Ottawa Prenatal Prospective Study.[58]

Most of the research on the teratogenicity of prenatal marijuana exposure has found no effect on morphology,[44,63-66] except Hingson and colleagues[62] reported an increased rate of minor physical anomalies as a result of prenatal marijuana use.

The relationship between prenatal marijuana exposure and neurobehavioral outcome is also uncertain.[57] Some authors[67] have reported effects of exposure on infant behavior using the Brazelton Neonatal Behavioral Assessment Scale, while others have not found significant effects.[60,61,68] At follow-up, Streissguth and associates[51] reported no association between prenatal marijuana use and IQ scores of four-year-olds, but Fried and Watkinson found that prenatally exposed (heavy use) four-year-olds had poorer memory skills than children of the moderate- or light-using mothers.[42] In a recent analysis, marijuana use during the first and second trimesters of pregnancy was associated with poorer performance on the Stanford-Binet Intelligence Scale composite score, short-term memory, verbal, and abstract-visual reasoning subscales.[69] These effects, particularly among the Caucasian offspring, were moderated by the child's attendance at preschool or day care.[69]

PRENATAL SUBSTANCE USE AND EFFECTS ON OFFSPRING OF ADOLESCENTS–PITTSBURGH STUDY

Previous research on the effects of prenatal exposure to various substances has focused on populations of adults and their offspring. In 1990, the first prospective study to examine the effects of prenatal substance use on the offspring of adolescents was conducted. This paper will report our findings from a cohort of adolescent mother/infant (live-born) dyads who participated in the study. Several of the citations which follow are from reports of earlier analyses of the cohort.

Methods

The 414 subjects were pregnant adolescents (18 years and younger) who attended the outpatient prenatal clinic at the Magee-Womens Hospital in Pittsburgh, PA, between 1990 and 1994, and their offspring. Data were collected at the end of the first trimester of pregnancy and at delivery. During the first interview, information was obtained on licit and illicit drug use covering the year prior to pregnancy and the first trimester. Second and third trimester drug use was included in the second interview. Information regarding demographic status, psychosocial and socioeconomic factors, and medical and sexual history was also collected at both times.

Infants were examined 24 to 36 hours after delivery by a trained pediatric nurse who was blind to maternal substance use. Crown-to-heel length and head and chest circumference were measured, and gestational age was assessed by physical exam.[70] Infants were examined for major and minor physical anomalies. Chart reviews were done on hospital deaths and on fetal deaths after 20 weeks' gestation. Birthweight and Apgar scores (one and five minutes) were transcribed from the medical record.

The measures of tobacco, marijuana, alcohol, and other substances used in the current study were developed to reflect accurately both the pattern and level of use, particularly during the first trimester.[71] In addition to quantity and frequency of substance use, information on age of onset of use and peer use was collected.

Sample Characteristics

The final cohort consisted of 414 teenagers who, on average, were 16.3 years old (range = 12-18). Sixty-nine percent were African-American; 31% were Caucasian. They had completed an average of 9.9 years of education (range = 6-13). Their average personal income was $85/month and the average family income was $891/month; only 19% were aware of their family income status. Ten (2.4%) of the teenagers were married by the time of delivery. At the initial interview, 63% were in school full-time and by the end of the third trimester, 57% were in school full-time. Many of the teens (71%) were living with a parent at the end of the first trimester, 10% lived with the father of the baby or a male friend, and 19% with another relative or friend, or in a group home. By the end of the third trimester, 62% were residing with at least one parent, 16% with the father of the baby or a male friend, and 22% with another relative or friend, or in a group home. Thirty-eight percent of the teenagers' mothers were also teenagers when they had their first child.

The current pregnancy was the first pregnancy for 74% of the subjects (mean gravidity = 1.25; range = 1-4). Nine percent had at least one spontaneous abortion and 7.3% had at least one elective abortion. The teenagers gained an average of 34 pounds during pregnancy (range = -31-110). The mean age of menarche was 11.9 years (range = 7-16) and first sexual intercourse was at 14.2 years (range = 9-17). Pregnancy was unplanned for 83%; 20% used birth control. Fifteen percent were breast feeding after delivery.

Fifty-one percent of the infants were male. The mean one and five minute Apgar scores were 8 (range = 1-9) and 8.8 (range = 1-10), respectively. The mean gestational age by sonar exam was 38.8 weeks (range = 23-43), and the mean birth weight was 3128.5 grams (range = 587-4863). Twelve percent of the infants were born prematurely (<37 weeks), 10% were LBW (<2500 gm), and 10% were small-for-gestational age (SGA).

Tobacco Use

In the year prior to pregnancy, 58% of the teenagers smoked cigarettes. This proportion dropped to 50% in the first trimester and then rose to 60% in the third trimester.[72] This increase was in sharp contrast to the decrease in marijuana and alcohol use among the teenagers[73] and the decrease in smoking, alcohol and marijuana use during pregnancy in the adult cohort.[32] The average number of cigarettes per day among the smokers was 7.6 (.5-30), 9.4 (.5-40), 8.0 (.33-30), and 7.6 (.5-30) for pre-pregnancy, first, second and third trimesters, respectively. Caucasian teenagers were significantly more likely to be smokers and to be heavier smokers than African-American teenagers. Seventy-nine percent of the Caucasians were smokers in the first trimester. This rate increased to 82% by the third trimester as compared to 52% in the African-American women. The most preferred brand of cigarettes was Newport (46%), followed by Marlboro (10%). Heavier tobacco users were more likely to drink alcohol and to use marijuana and cocaine. They had more friends who smoked, drank, and used marijuana than light or non-smokers.[72]

Thirty-eight percent of the adolescents abstained from tobacco throughout pregnancy. Of the 62% who smoked at some time in their pregnancy, 57% either smoked at the same level throughout pregnancy, increased quantity or initiated smoking. The remaining 43% of the smokers decreased the quantity of smoking or quit.[72]

Prenatal Tobacco Effects on Infant Outcome

We examined the effects of prenatal tobacco exposure during each trimester on the newborns using regression analyses.[74] The covariates were: race, infant sex, maternal age, maternal height, pre-pregnancy weight, pregnancy weight gain, adequacy of prenatal care, maternal nutrition, gravidity, household structure, social support, teenager's parent's education, school status, alcohol use, and marijuana, cocaine/crack and other illicit drug use. Effects with $p \leq .05$ were considered to be statistically significant. First trimester tobacco use significantly predicted decreased birthweight and head circumference by 10.1 gm/cigarette and .32 mm/cigarette, respectively. This is a reduction of 202 gm in birthweight and 6.4 mm in head circumference for each pack per day. Second trimester tobacco use reduced birth length by .34 mm/cigarette or 6.8 mm/ pack/day.

In the study of an adult cohort who attended the same prenatal clinic as the adolescent cohort, prenatal tobacco use effects on infant growth were significant but not as large.[32] Birthweight was reduced by 158 grams per pack/day and head circumference by 2.8 mm/pack/day. First trimester smoking reduced birth length by 6.4 mm/pack/day.

Alcohol Use

Seventy-four percent of the adolescents were drinking in the year prior to pregnancy. This rate dropped to 47%, 12% and 8% in the first, second, and third trimesters, respectively. Heavier drinkers were more likely to be Caucasian, were more likely to report that they meant to be pregnant and that they recognized their pregnancy later than light or non-drinkers. Heavier drinkers were more likely to smoke and to use marijuana and cocaine. They had more friends who used tobacco and marijuana than light or non-drinkers and were less likely to live with their parents and to be in school full-time.

In a comparison of drinking patterns between teenagers and adults who attended the same prenatal clinic, binge drinking (5+ drinks/day) was more common in adults (39%) than teenagers (31%) prior to pregnancy. However, in the first trimester, binge drinking increased to 37% among the teenagers and fell to 27% among the adults. Caucasian teenagers had the highest rates of binge drinking (51%), followed by African-American teenagers (27%), Caucasian adults (23%) and African-American adults (20%).[73,75]

Prenatal Alcohol Effects on Infant Outcome

We examined the effects of prenatal alcohol exposure during each trimester using linear regression analyses. The covariates were: race, infant sex, maternal age, maternal height, pre-pregnancy weight, pregnancy weight gain, adequacy of prenatal care, maternal nutrition, gravidity, household structure, social support, teenager's parent's education, school status, and use of marijuana, tobacco, cocaine/crack and other illicit drug use. After controlling for the above covariates, second trimester alcohol use was significantly associated with a decrease in gestational age of 7 days per drink per day. After controlling for gestational age, second trimester alcohol (any) use also significantly reduced birthweight (117 grams) and head circumference (5 mm). In addition, second trimester alcohol exposure significantly reduced one-minute and five-minute Apgar scores, on average, by .5 points and .2 points, respectively. Using logistic regression analysis, we found that second trimester alcohol use increased the probability of LBW by 2.4 times.

We found significant racial differences in prenatal drinking patterns so we analyzed the data separately by race. Alcohol use has a greater average impact on reducing birthweight and head circumference in Caucasians as compared to African-Americans (311 gm vs. 142 gm; 10 mm vs. 6 mm, respectively). Alcohol, however, had a larger effect on the probability of LBW in African-Americans than in Caucasians (odds ratios = 2.5 and 1.4, respectively). Alcohol use significantly reduced gestational age in African-Americans (7 days/drink/day), but did not significantly affect gestational age among Caucasians. First trimester alcohol use increased the risk of 3+ minor physical anomalies in African-Americans (odds ratio = 2.2).

In contrast, prenatal alcohol use did not significantly predict gestational age or birthweight in the newborn offspring of the adults who attended the same prenatal clinic.[43] Only head circumference was affected by alcohol use in the first and second months of the first trimester. Drinking at the rate of one or more drinks/day was found to reduce infant head circumference on average by .64 mm.

Marijuana Use

In the year prior to pregnancy, 36.5% of the teenagers used marijuana. This rate dropped to 16.5% in the first trimester, and to 4.9% and 2.9% in the second and third trimesters, respectively. Marijuana use was significantly related to earlier age of first sexual intercourse and earlier age onset of tobacco and alcohol use. Those who used marijuana were less likely to be in school full-time, less likely to attend church regularly, and were more depressed. Those who were heavy users of marijuana (1+ joints per day) were also heavy tobacco and alcohol users and were more likely to binge drink (drink 5+ drinks per occasion). Among the marijuana users, the average daily joints per day was .87 (.0025-20.0), .72 (.01-8.0), .23 (.01-8.0), and .26 (.01-8.0) in the year before pregnancy, first, second, and third trimesters, respectively.

The teenagers exhibited the expected progression in the onset of substance use with age. The mean ages of onset of tobacco, alcohol, marijuana and cocaine/crack use were 13.4, 13.6, 14.4 and 14.9 years, respectively. Sexual activity began at an average age of 14.2 years.

Prenatal Marijuana Effects on Infant Outcome

We examined the effects of marijuana use on neonatal outcome using the same analyses as those described above.[74] The covariates were the same except that the covariate tobacco use replaced marijuana use. The variable "average daily joints per day" (ADJ) significantly predicted reduced gestational age by 9 days/joint/day. ADJ did not predict any of the growth or morphology outcomes. Because there were only fifteen and nine users in the second and third trimesters, respectively, we ran the regressions with the marijuana variable dichotomized as user/non-user. After controlling for covariates described earlier, first trimester marijuana use (any) was significantly associated with a decrease in gestational age of 7 days. Using logistic regression analysis, we found that second trimester marijuana use (any) increased the risk of small-for-gestational age by three-fold. Among Caucasians, first trimester marijuana use (any) increased the probability of minor physical anomalies (odds ratio = 3.2).

In the adult study, marijuana use predicted decreased birth length by 1.5 mm using the dichotomous variable 1+ joints per day/non-users.[44] Marijuana use did not predict any other birth outcome.

COMMENT ON THE PITTSBURGH ADOLESCENT FINDINGS

Tobacco, alcohol and marijuana use were very common in the cohort of pregnant teenagers. These teenagers were three times more likely to smoke than non-pregnant high school seniors in a national sample in 1992.[3] This is of particular concern given the 1990 Health Objectives for the Nation which stated that "The proportion of women who smoke during pregnancy should be no greater than one-half the proportion of women overall who smoke."[76] Similarly, the annual prevalence of marijuana use in the year prior to becoming pregnant among our teenagers of 37% was considerably higher than the annual prevalence of use of 26% among seniors reported in the national study.[3]

We found that those adolescent mothers who smoked tobacco during pregnancy were also more likely to drink, to binge on alcohol in the first trimester, and to use illicit drugs. Mothers who smoked heavily had significantly lower pre-pregnancy weight, a risk factor for LBW, than those who were light smokers or non-smokers. In addition, later recognition of pregnancy was a significant correlate of heavier tobacco use. Similarly, teens who used marijuana were more likely to drink alcohol and binge drink in early pregnancy, and heavier marijuana users smoked more cigarettes and drank more alcohol. Binge drinking and later recognition of pregnancy both occurred in the crucial period of organogenesis in the first trimester.[77] Teenagers who both binged on alcohol and recognized pregnancy later also smoked more heavily in the third trimester, the period of most rapid fetal growth. These observations highlight the importance of considering the cumulative effect of risk factors in the fetus of the mother who uses tobacco, alcohol, and/or marijuana.

Although marijuana, alcohol and other illicit drug use dropped considerably in the first trimester, tobacco use among the teenagers actually increased during pregnancy, from 50% to 60% between the first and third trimesters. This also contrasts with the relatively constant rates of smoking during pregnancy, 54% in trimester one and 53% in trimester three, in the adult cohort.[32] The increase in smoking during pregnancy among the teenagers is disturbing. The benefits that may be derived from the reduction in the use of other substances may be offset by the increase in tobacco use. Although the messages about negative fetal effects from substances other than tobacco seem to be reaching pregnant teenagers, these young women need to be educated about the effects of prenatal tobacco use on the offspring. Evidence suggests that if a woman stops smoking early in pregnancy her risk of delivering a LBW infant approaches that of a non-smoker.[78] Consequently, smoking cessation programs should be offered at the initial prenatal visit. Teens commonly turn to peers as role models.[79] Because we found peer tobacco, alcohol, and marijuana use to be strong and consistent predictors of prenatal use of these substances, it might be advantageous to utilize some type of peer support mechanism in any intervention.

Our analyses demonstrated a significant relationship between prenatal tobacco use and infant size at birth after controlling for other substance use and multiple covariates. At birth, weight, length, head and chest circumferences, and Ponderal index were all negatively associated with tobacco exposure. Prenatal tobacco exposure did not affect gestational age, or rates of prematurity and SGA, but it did significantly increase the rate of LBW among African-American offspring.

Second trimester alcohol use was significantly associated with a decrease in gestational age. After controlling for gestational age, second trimester alcohol (any) use also significantly reduced birthweight and head circumference. In addition, second trimester alcohol exposure significantly reduced one-minute and five-minute Apgar scores. Second trimester alcohol use increased the probability of low birth weight by 2.4 times.

First trimester marijuana use was associated with reduced gestational age in the total cohort, and an increase in minor physical anomalies among the Caucasian offspring. Prenatal marijuana use did not significantly affect infant size. Interpretations of our findings on the effects of prenatal marijuana use among adolescents are limited due to the low level of exposure. Although many of the teenagers used marijuana prior to getting pregnant, only 17% were using marijuana in the first trimester, and this rate and level dropped precipitously in the second and third trimesters. Despite this low exposure level, first trimester use was significantly associated with reduced gestational age.

Overall, the prevalence of prenatal tobacco, alcohol and marijuana use was high among these adolescents, although the quantity of use was low. Nevertheless, effects on the offspring of reduced gestational age and size were still evident. It should be noted that the average reduction in any specific growth parameter was modest in magnitude; however, when considering the reduction of gestational age of one week in a population already at high risk for prematurity, and a reduction in neonatal size in a population already at high risk for lower birth weight, these effects take on added significance. These negative effects may be further moderated as the child continues to develop physically, socially, and emotionally in a postnatal environment that has been described as less-than-optimal. At the time of this report, no study has examined the long-term effects of prenatal tobacco, alcohol and marijuana use on growth, cognitive or behavioral outcomes of the offspring of adolescent mothers. Future research studies are warranted to examine the interrelationships and interaction of the prenatal and postnatal environments of the children of adolescents.

REFERENCES

1. National Center for Health Statistics. Advance Report of the Final Natality Statistics, 1991. *Monthly Vital Statistics Report*, Hyattsville, MD: Author, Supplement 42(3); 1993.

2. Centers for Disease Control. Youth Risk Behavior Survey, Selected behaviors that increase the risk for HIV infection among high school students-United States, 1991. MMWR 1992;41:945-950.

3. Johnston L, O'Malley P, Bachman J. National survey results on drug use from monitoring the future study, 1975-1992. Rockville, MD: NIDA, NIH Pub. No. 13-3597; 1994.

4. Zuckerman B, Alpert J, Dooling E. Neonatal outcome: Is adolescent pregnancy a risk factor? *Pediatr.* 1983;71:489-493.

5. Babsin S, Clark M. Relationships between infant death and maternal age. *J Pediatr.* 1983;103:391-393.

6. Hechtman L. Teenage mothers and their children: Risks and problems: A review. *Can J Psychiatr.* 1989;34:569-575.

7. Hofferth S. The effects of programs and policies on adolescent pregnancy and childbearing. In: Hayes C ed. *Risking the Future, Vol. 1.* Washington, DC: Natl Acad Press; 1987.

8. Furstenberg F, Levine J, Brooks-Gunn J. The children of teenage mothers: Patterns of early childbearing in two generations. *Fam Plann Perspect.* 1990;22:54-61.

9. Moore K, Snyder N. *Cognitive Development Among the Children of Adolescent Mothers.* Washington, DC: Child Trends, Inc; 1990.

10. Maracek J. Economic, Social, and Psychological Consequences of Adolescent Childbearing: An Analysis of Data from the Philadelphia Collaborative Perinatal Project. *Final Report to the National Institute of Child Health and Human Development.* Philadelphia, PA: Institute for the Continuous Study of Man, 1979.

11. Chase-Landsdale L, Brooks-Gunn J, Paikoff R. Research and programs for adolescent mothers: Missing links and future promises. *Fam Rel.* 1991;40:396-403.

12. Benn R, Salts E. The effects of grandmother support on teen parenting and infant attachment patterns within the family. Paper presented at the meeting of the *Society for Research on Child Development*, Kansas City, MO, 1989.

13. Moran D, Whitman T. The multiple effects of a play oriented parent training program for mothers of developmentally delayed children. *Analysis and Intervention in Developmental Disabilities.* 1985;5:73-96.

14. Naeye R. Influence of maternal cigarette smoking during pregnancy on fetal and childhood growth. *Obstet Gynecol.* 1981;57:18-21.

15. Zuckerman B, Walker D, Frank D, Chase C. Adolescent pregnancy and parenthood. *Advances Dev Behav Pediatr.* 1986;7:275-311.

16. Whitman T, Borkowski J, Schnellenbach C, Nath P. Predicting and understanding developmental delay of children of adolescent mothers: A multi-dimensional approach. *Am J of Mental Deficiency.* 1987;92:40-56.

17. Black C, DeBlassie E. Adolescent pregnancy: Contributing factors, consequences, treatment and plausible solutions. *Adolesc.* 1985;78:281-290.

18. Zuckerman B, Walker D, Frank D, Chase C, Hamburg B. Adolescent pregnancy biobehavioral determinants of outcome. *J Pediatr.* 1984;105:857-863.

19. Ketterilinus R. Maternal age, socio-demographics, prenatal health and behavior: Influences on neonatal risk status. *J Adolesc Health Care.* 1990;11:423-431.

20. Garcia-Coll C, Hoffman J, Oh W. The social context of teenage childbearing: Effects on the infant's care-giving environment. *J Youth Adolesc.* 1987;6:345-360.

21. Sadler L, Catrone C. The adolescent parent: A dual developmental crisis. *J Adolesc Health Care.* 1983;4:100-105.

22. Pandina R, Schuele J. Psychosocial correlates of alcohol and drug use of adolescent students and adolescents in treatment. *J Stud Alc.* 1983;44:950-973.

23. McCubbin H, Patterson J. Adolescent stress, coping and adaptation: A normative family perspective. In: Leigh GK, Peterson GW eds. *Adolescence in a Family Context.* Cincinnati, OH: South-Western Publishers; 1986: 256-276.

24. Codega S, Pasley B, Kreutzer J. Coping behaviors of adolescent mothers: An exploratory study and comparison of Mexican-Americans and Anglos. *J Adol Res.* 1990;5:34-53.

25. Zuckerman B, Amaro H, Beardslee W. Mental health of adolescent mothers: The implications of depression and drug use. *J Dev Behav Pediatr.* 1987;8:111-116.

26. Kaplan S, Landan B, Weinhold C. Adverse health behaviors and depressive symptomatology in adolescents. *J Am Acad Child Psychiatr.* 1984;233:595-601.

27. Colletta N. At risk for depression: A study of young mothers. *J Genet Psychol.* 1983;142:301-310.

28. Donovan J, Jessor R. Adolescent problem drinking, psychosocial correlates in a national sample study. *J Stud Alc.* 1978;38:1506-1524.

29. Hundleby J, Carpenter R, Ross R. Adolescent drug use and other behaviors. *J Child Psychol Psychiatr.* 1982;23:61-68.

30. Pletsch P. Substance use and health activities of pregnant adolescents. *J Adolesc Health Care.* 1988;9:38-45.

31. Kline J, Stein Z, Hutzler M. Cigarettes, alcohol and marijuana: Varying associations with birthweight. *Int J Epidemiol.* 1987;16:44-51.

32. Day N, Cornelius M, Goldschmidt L, Richardson G, Robles N, Taylor P. The effects of prenatal tobacco and marijuana use on offspring growth from birth through age 3 years. *Neurotoxicol Teratol.* 1992;14:407-414.

33. Persson P, Grennert L, Gennser G, Kullander S. A study of smoking and pregnancy with special reference to fetal growth. *Acta Obstet et Gynecol Scand.* 1978;78:33-39.

34. Rantakallio P. A follow-up study up to age 14 of children whose mothers smoked during pregnancy. *Acta Pediatr Scand.* 1983;72:747-753.

35. Fogelman K, Manor O. Smoking in pregnancy and development into early adulthood. *Brit Med J.* 1988;297:1233-1236.

36. Fried P, O'Connell. A comparison of the effects of prenatal exposure to tobacco, alcohol cannabis and caffeine on birth size and subsequent growth. *Neurotoxicol Teratol.* 1987;19:79-85.

37. Hardy J, Mellits E. Does maternal smoking during pregnancy have a long term effect on the child? *Lancet.* 1972;2:1332-1336.

38. Himmelburger D, Brown B, Cohen E. Cigarette smoking during pregnancy and the occurrence of spontaneous abortion and congenital abnormality. *Am J Epid.* 1978;108:470-479.

39. Malloy M, Kleinman J, Land G, Schramm W. The association of maternal smoking with age and cause of infant death. *Am J Epidemiol.* 1988;128:46-55.

40. Kristjansson E, Fried P, Watkinson B. Maternal smoking during pregnancy affects children's vigilance performance. *Drug Alcohol Depend.* 1989;24:11-19.

41. Fried P, Watkinson B. 12- and 24-month neurobehavioral follow-up of children prenatally exposed to marijuana, cigarettes and alcohol. *Neurotoxicol Teratol.* 1988;10:305-313.

42. Fried P, Watkinson B. 36- and 48-month neurobehavioral follow-up of children prenatally exposed to marijuana, cigarettes and alcohol. *Neurotoxicol Teratol.* 1990;11:49.

43. Day N, Jasperse D, Richardson G, Robles N, Sambamoorthi U, Taylor P, Scher M, Stoffer D, Bloom M. Prenatal exposure to alcohol: Effect on infant growth and morphologic characteristics. *Pediatr.* 1989;84:536-541.

44. Day N, Sambamoorthi U, Taylor P, Richardson G, Robles N, Jhon Y, Scher M, Stoffer D, Cornelius M, Jasperse D. Prenatal marijuana use and neonatal outcome. *Neurotoxicol Teratol.* 1991;13:329-334.

45. Lemoine P, Harrousseau H, Borteyru J, Menuet J. Children of alcoholic parents. Abnormalities observed in 127 cases. *Quest Med.* 1968;21:476-482.

46. Jones K, Smith D. Recognition of the fetal alcohol syndrome in early infancy. *Lancet,* 1973, 2:999-1001.

47. Golden N, Sokol R, Kuhnert B, Bottoms S. Maternal alcohol use and infant development. *Pediatr.* 1982;70:931-934.

48. Graham J, Hanson J, Darby B, Barr H, Streissguth A. Independent dysmorphology evaluations at birth and 4 years of age for children exposed to varying amounts of alcohol in utero. *Pediatr.* 1988;81:772-778.

49. Steinhausen H, Nestler V, Spohr H. Development and psycho-pathology of children with fetal alcohol syndrome. *J Dev Behav Pediatr.* 1982;3:49-54.

50. Streissguth A, Aase J, Clarren S, Randels S, LaDue R, Smith D. Fetal alcohol syndrome in adolescents and adults. *J Am Med Assoc.* 1991;265:1961-1967.

51. Streissguth A, Sampson P, Barr H. In: Hutchings DE ed. Prenatal Abuse of Licit and Illicit Drugs. *Ann NY Acad Sci.* 1989;562:145-158.

52. Day N, Richardson G, Robles N, Sambamoorthi U, Taylor P, Scher M, Stoffer D, Jasperse D, Cornelius M. The effect of prenatal alcohol exposure on growth and morphology of the offspring at 8 months of age. *Pediatr.* 1990;85:748-752.

53. Day N, Richardson G, Robles N, Goldschmidt L, Taylor P, Cornelius M, Scher M. Prenatal alcohol exposure and offspring growth at 18 months of age: The predictive validity of two measures of drinking. *Alc Clin Exp Res.* 1991;15:914-918.

54. Day N, Robles N, Richardson G, Geva D, Taylor P, Scher M, Stoffer D, Cornelius M, Goldschmidt L. The effects of prenatal alcohol use on the growth of children at three years of age. *Alc Clin Exp Res.* 1991;15:67-71.

55. Brown R, Coles C, Smith I, Platzman K, Silverstein J, Erickson S, Falek A. Effects of prenatal alcohol exposure at school age. II. Attention and behavior. *Neurotoxicol Teratol.* 1991;13:369-376.

56. Coles D, Brown R, Smith I, Platzman K, Erickson S, Falek A. Effects of prenatal alcohol exposure at school age. I. Physical and Cognitive Development. *Neurotox Teratol.* 1991;13:357-367.

57. Richardson G, Day N, McGaughey P. The impact of prenatal marijuana and cocaine use on the infant and child. In: Woods J ed. *Clinical Obstetrics and Gynecology.* 1993;36:302-318.

58. Fried P, Watkinson B, Willan A. Marijuana use during pregnancy and decreased length of gestation. *Am J Obstet Gynecol.* 1984;150:23.

59. Hatch E, Bracken M. Effect of marijuana use in pregnancy on fetal growth. *Am J Epidemiol.* 1986;124:986.

60. Tennes K, Avitable N, Backard C, Boyles C, Hassoun B, Holmes L, Kreye M. Marijuana: Prenatal and postnatal exposure in the human. In: Pinkert T ed. *NIDA Res Monogr.* 1985;59:48-62.

61. Hayes J, Dreher M, Nugent J. Newborn outcomes with maternal marihuana use in Jamaican women. *Ped Nursing.* 1988;14:107.

62. Hingson R, Alpert J, Day N, Dooling E, Kayne H, Morelock S, Oppenheimer E, Zuckerman B. Effects of maternal drinking and marijuana use on fetal growth and development. *Pediatr.* 1982;70:539-546.

63. Linn S, Shoenbaum S, Monson R, Rosner R, Stubblefield P, Ryan K. The association of marijuana use with outcome of pregnancy. *Am J Pub Hlth.* 1983;73:1161-1174.

64. Zuckerman B, Frank D, Hingson R, Amaro H, Levenson S, Kayne H, Parker S, Vinci R, Aboagye K, Fried L, Cabral H, Timperi R, Baucher H. Effects of maternal marijuana and cocaine use on fetal growth. *N Engl J Med.* 1989;320:762-768.

65. Astley S, Clarren S, Little R, Sampson P, Daling J. Analysis of facial shape in children gestationally exposed to marijuana, alcohol, and/or cocaine. *Pediatr.* 1992;89:67.

66. O'Connell C, Fried P. An investigation of prenatal cannabis exposure and minor physical anomalies in a low risk population. *Neurobehav Toxicol Teratol.* 1984;6:345-350.

67. Fried P, Makin J. Neonatal behavioural correlates of prenatal exposure to marihuana, cigarettes and alcohol in a low risk population. *Neurotoxicol Teratol.* 1987;9(1):1-7.

68. Richardson G, Day N, Taylor P. The effect of prenatal alcohol, marijuana and tobacco exposure on neonatal behavior. *Inf Beh Dev* 1989;12:199.

69. Day N, Richardson G, Goldschmidt L, Robles N, Taylor P, Stoffer D, Cornelius M, Geva D. The effect of prenatal marijuana exposure on the cognitive development of offspring at age three. *Neurotoxicol Teratol.* 1994;16(2):169-175.

70. Ballard J, Novak K, Driver M. A simplified score for assessment of fetal maturation of newly born infants. *Pediatr.* 1979;95:769-774.

71. Day N, Robles N. Methodological issues in the measurement of substance use. In: Hutchings D ed. Prenatal Abuse of Licit and Illicit Drugs. *Ann NY Acad Sci.* 1989;562:8-13.

72. Cornelius M, Geva D, Day N, Cornelius J, Taylor P. Patterns and covariates of tobacco use in a recent sample of pregnant teenagers. *J Adol Hlth.* 1994;15:528-535.

73. Cornelius M, Day N, Cornelius J, Taylor P, Geva D, Richardson G. Drinking patterns and correlates of drinking among pregnant teenagers. *Alc Clin Exp Res.* 1993;17(2):290-294.

74. Cornelius M, Taylor P, Geva D, Day N. Prenatal tobacco and marijuana use among adolescents: Effects on offspring Gestational Age, Growth and Morphology. *Pediatr.* 1995;95:738-743.

75. Cornelius M, Richardson G, Day N, Cornelius J, Geva D, Taylor P. A comparison of prenatal drinking in two recent samples of teenagers and adults. *J Stud Alc.* 1994;55:412-419.

76. U.S. Department of Health and Human Services. *Healthy People 2000: National Health Promotion and Disease Prevention Objectives.* DHHS Publication No. PHS91-50213. Washington, DC: Government Printing Office;1991.

77. Vorhees C. Concepts in teratology and developmental toxicology derived from animal research. In: Hutchings D ed. *Ann NY Acad Sci.* 1989;562:31-41.

78. Alexander L. The pregnant smoker: Nursing implications. *J Obstet Gynec Neonatal Nurs.* 1987;16:167-173.

79. Duffy J, Coates T. Reducing smoking among pregnant adolescents. *Adolescence.* 1989;24:29-37.

Fetal Cocaine Exposure: Neurologic Effects and Sensory-Motor Delays

Robert E. Arendt
Sonnia Minnes
Lynn T. Singer

SUMMARY. Research on animal models demonstrates that fetal cocaine exposure results in neurologic deficits in memory and learning. Although drug effects on human infants are difficult to separate from other environmental influences of a drug-using lifestyle, studies suggest that infants exposed to cocaine in utero have reduced growth, delays in sensory-motor development, attentional deficits, and depressed responsivity to social stimulation. Standard interventions to promote behavioral state regulation in affected infants may be helpful when parents are capable of participating. *[Article copies available from The Haworth Document Delivery Service: 1-800-342-9678. E-mail address: getinfo@haworth.com]*

The history of research on the effects of in utero cocaine exposure has been both short and turbulent. In the 10 years since the "crack baby" was

Robert E. Arendt, PhD, Sonnia Minnes, and Lynn T. Singer are affiliated with the Department of Pediatrics, Case Western Reserve University, School of Medicine, Cleveland, OH.

Address correspondence to Robert E. Arendt, Department of Pediatrics, Division of Pediatric Psychology and Speech and Language, 11100 Euclid Avenue, Cleveland, OH 44106.

This research was supported by Grants number R29-DA07358 and R01-DA07957 from the National Institute for Drug Abuse and Grant RR00080 from the General Clinical Research Center.

[Haworth co-indexing entry note]: "Fetal Cocaine Exposure: Neurologic Effects and Sensory-Motor Delays." Arendt, Robert E., Sonnia Minnes, and Lynn T. Singer. Co-published simultaneously in *Physical & Occupational Therapy in Pediatrics* (The Haworth Press, Inc.) Vol. 16, No. 1/2, 1996, pp. 129-144; and: *Children with Prenatal Drug Exposure* (ed: Lynette S. Chandler, and Shelly J. Lane) The Haworth Press, Inc., 1996, pp. 129-144. Single or multiple copies of this article are available from The Haworth Document Delivery Service [1-800-342-9678, 9:00 a.m. - 5:00 p.m. (EST). E-mail address: getinfo@haworth.com].

© 1996 by The Haworth Press, Inc. All rights reserved.

first identified and birth outcomes reported, findings have been controversial and at times contradictory. Perinatal epidemiologic studies in the late 1980s documented the large numbers of infants born after fetal exposure to cocaine. Estimates of the proportion of babies born in urban teaching hospitals who test positive for cocaine range from 5-45%.[1-4] Early alarming reports about pronounced neurobehavioral abnormalities in neonates exposed to cocaine in utero[5-7] raised subsequent concerns about potential long-term neurodevelopmental effects on fetal and infant outcome. Recent reports, however, indicate that the effects may be subtle and could be masked and/or confounded by environmental factors, such as amount of prenatal care[8] or socioeconomic status.[9]

Part of the ambiguity in results might be attributed to the initial lack of information regarding effects of cocaine on human development. With little else to go on, investigators interested in studying the effects of cocaine on the human fetus had two potential bodies of research on which to draw, the known effects of cocaine on adults and on animals. As the volume of literature grew, several issues central to the further study of prenatal exposure to a potentially neurotoxic agent became evident: (a) whether any pre- or perinatal neurologic effect could be attributed to cocaine, (b) whether identified effects could be related to specific neurobehavioral outcomes, and (c) the long-term consequences. An examination, therefore, of the evidence pertaining to the neurologic development of infants exposed to cocaine follows. Additionally, some considerations concerning intervention are offered.

RATIONALE FOR STUDYING THE NEUROLOGIC EFFECTS OF FETAL COCAINE EXPOSURE

Cocaine's central and peripheral nervous system effects on adults have been widely recognized, thus raising questions regarding a potential teratogenic effect. Cocaine easily crosses the placental barrier during gestation.[10] In particular, central nervous system (CNS) alteration during gestation secondary to cocaine exposure[11] could result in long-term functional deficits manifesting in behavioral and cognitive abnormalities.

In adults, cocaine use has been related to cerebrovascular accidents,[12,13] high blood pressure, and seizures.[14] Cocaine's known actions on several neurotransmitter systems in the mature adult have been well-defined.[15] Cocaine acts to prevent re-uptake of catecholamines presynaptically, resulting in an increased level of these neurotransmitters. Alterations in catecholamine levels during fetal gestation may affect the maturation of fetal neurotransmitter systems.[16,17] Maternal cocaine use also results in concomitant rise in maternal blood pressure as a result of vasoconstriction and tachycardia, decreasing uterine and placental blood flow.[11] This interference with blood flow to the fetus reduces oxygen supply and may cause chronic hypoxia which interferes with normal CNS development.

EVIDENCE FOR NEUROLOGIC EFFECT

Animal Studies

The animal literature to date supports the notion that fetal cocaine exposure has deleterious effects on neurological outcome and subsequent neurobehavioral competence. Disruptions in neuro- and gliogenesis and alterations in brain metabolism, especially in opiate and cholinergic systems, are reported.[18] Gestational cocaine exposure in rats has been associated with cephalic hemorrhages, eye abnormalities, and cortical and brainstem defects.[19,20]

Deficits in classical conditioning, an early form of learning, and difficulties in learning tasks such as maze performance and operant learning trials, have also been reported in animal studies, suggesting that cocaine may function as a behavioral teratogen with long-term effects on functional abilities later in life. Animal studies have demonstrated that cocaine exposure in fetal rats adversely affects areas of the brain important for memory and learning, for the regulation of movement and growth, and for reproductive function.[21] Learning systems in animals may be differentially affected by cocaine exposure as well. Cocaine-treated rat pups have shown learning and retention difficulties using conditioning models,[22,23] although not all studies have demonstrated deficits.[24]

Animal studies allow the isolation of specific effects of fetal cocaine exposure apart from the confounds inherent in human populations, such as polydrug use, poverty, or poor nutrition. Unfortunately, findings from animal studies are not necessarily generalizable to human populations. Spear points out, however, that results of human clinical studies of neurotoxicants generally correspond closely to those of laboratory animal studies when similar outcome behaviors are assessed.[18] Thus, it would be highly atypical if the effects of cocaine exposure found in animal studies did not also occur in humans. Spear's conclusion from a review of available animal studies on the behavioral consequences of gestational cocaine exposure is that data to date provide "convincing evidence that cocaine is a behavioral teratogen in animal models."[18]

Human Studies

Human studies addressing the neurologic effects of cocaine on the fetus and subsequent development have also been emerging. Volpe[25] presented a convincing summary of some of the potential mechanisms of destructive neural effects secondary to fetal cocaine exposure, noting that the genesis of CNS effects is likely to be multifactorial. In any case, the neurologic system is significantly affected by fetal hypoxemia caused by impaired placental blood flow resulting in impaired fetal cerebrovascular autoregulation. Such impairments make the fetal brain highly vulnerable to changes in blood pressure, including hemorrhages in the immediate neonatal period. Constriction of blood vessels after cocaine exposure, a well-documented effect in animals, decreases nourishment to the fetus and reduces brain growth.

Recent reports have suggested significant CNS effects in newborns who were exposed to cocaine during gestation in addition to obstetric complications.[1,2,26] Microcephaly, an abnormality reflecting impairment in intrauterine brain growth (defined as head circumference more than 2 SD below the mean), has been widely reported in cohorts of cocaine-exposed neonates.[27,28,29] The prominence of microcephaly, an index of brain size, in cocaine-exposed infants, has been construed as one marker of its CNS effects because of its association with later developmental delay. Reduced head size has been identified as a major predictor of depressed cognitive functioning following cocaine exposure.[30] Other electrophysiological alterations have been noted. These include seizure activity,[31] EEG abnormalities,[32] sleep discordance,[33] and abnormal brainstem conduction time.[34]

Serious destructive lesions suggesting prenatally occurring insults were reported in a series of case studies.[35-37] A San Diego study reported an 8-fold increase in cranial ultrasound abnormalities in term infants exposed to cocaine, a finding which was replicated in a Boston study.[38] The latter study also found a significant increase in risk for caudate echodensities in term infants who had been heavily exposed to cocaine during gestation when compared with lightly exposed or non-exposed infants,[38] a finding among the first to suggest a dose-response effect. Neurologic sequelae have also been found in cohorts of very low birthweight (VLBW) infants exposed to cocaine. One prospective study of 323 infants weighing less than 1500 grams at birth[39] reported a three-fold increase in the occurrence of seizures, among other medical problems, in infants exposed to cocaine. In our own studies of a sample of 41 infants exposed to cocaine, increased incidence of mild (Grade I and II) intraventricular hemorrhage was found at birth compared to controls matched for race, social class, and presence of bronchopulmonary dysplasia.[40]

Finally, numerous studies have employed the Brazelton Neonatal Behavioral Assessment Scale (BNBAS) to assess the neurobehavioral sequelae in the first month of life. Findings have been widely divergent and sometimes contradictory.[41] Several studies have reported depressed interactive behavior, impaired responses to environmental stimuli, and deficits in orientation, and in motor and state regulation in cocaine exposed cohorts. Other well designed studies, however, found no significant deficits on the BNBAS.

SENSORY-MOTOR DEVELOPMENT

The most serious consequences of an association between prenatal cocaine exposure and the many atypical neurologic effects reported may not be the rare cases of dramatic medical outcomes, but rather the insidious and likely much more widespread deleterious effects on long-term behavior and development. Delays in language development,[42] increased rates of behavior disorders,[43] and late acquisition of motor milestones[44] have all been suspected as possible negative consequences of prenatal cocaine exposure. Among other problems, laboratory studies of rats have found that early exposure to cocaine has later developmental effects on the functioning of the dopamine system,[18] particularly in areas of the brain involved in motor functioning.[45]

The importance of motor skills in any at-risk infant population, particularly one exposed to a possible teratogen, is often inferred from general findings suggesting that motor and perceptual skills, as opposed to verbal and symbolic skills, have a large biologic basis and are related to environmental factors in a less direct manner or to a lesser extent.[46] Additionally, early reflex and motor behavior is viewed as an early indicator of neurologic maturation. Several investigators chose, therefore, to study early motor development in infants exposed to cocaine.

One of the first studies to describe the development of these infants used the Movement Assessment of Infants (MAI).[47] The MAI has been employed in several subsequent studies to assess the early motoric development of at-risk infants. This measure provides a detailed and systematic appraisal of motor development during the first year. The MAI assesses muscle tone, primitive reflexes, automatic reactions, and volitional movements. Schneider and associates[48,49] tested 30 full term 4-month-olds exposed to cocaine and compared their scores on the MAI with scores from 50 infants selected from a convenience sample without drug exposure. The two groups differed significantly on the total risk score and on the muscle tone, reflexes, and volitional movements subscales. Schneider[49] concluded that, although in utero cocaine exposure does not have a significant effect on the motor development of all exposed infants, it appears to have a profound impact on some.

Rose-Jacobs and colleagues[50] also reported results using the MAI to compare cocaine-exposed and non-exposed infants at 4 months of age. Term infants participating in this study were classified as either heavier cocaine-exposed (n = 27), lighter cocaine-exposed (n = 61), or unexposed (n = 82). Using a regression model, an overall cocaine effect was found only in the volitional movements subscale. The more heavily exposed infants had significantly poorer mean scores then either the more lightly exposed or the unexposed. The authors concluded that their findings supported the importance of evaluating dose response to cocaine.

Arendt and colleagues[51] reported results of a study of sensory-motor development in 100 4-month-olds, 42 of whom were prenatally exposed to cocaine. Testers were masked as to drug status of infants. Overall scores from the MAI indicated a significant mean group difference, with the infants exposed to cocaine performing less well. The mean total score of the cocaine exposed group exceeded the high-risk cutoff score, suggesting that a significant percentage of the infants were at risk for motor delays.

In the same study, results from the Test of Sensory Functioning in Infants (TSFI) also revealed a significant difference between the groups. The TSFI is designed to assess sensory processing and reactivity in 4- to 18-month-olds. It evaluates response to tactile deep-pressure, visual-tactile integration, adaptive motor, ocular motor, and reactivity to vestibular stimulation. Again, the exposed group of infants performed significantly below the unexposed group, although mean scores of both groups were within the normal range.

Seventy of the children seen at 4 months (33 cocaine-exposed, 37 non-exposed) have been reassessed at 12 months of age using the Bayley Scales of Infant Development.[52] Preliminary results indicated that the cocaine-exposed group performed, on average, more poorly on the Motor Scale, but are still, as a group, performing within normal limits. There was no significant difference between groups on the Mental Scale.

A series of standard multiple regressions were conducted to determine whether early sensory-motor scores would predict later mental and motor scores. Results of these analyses suggested that the MAI total score, but not the TSFI total score, accounted for a significant portion of the variance in both Bayley Mental and Motor scores, even after accounting for gestational age. Further analysis revealed that the relationship between Bayley and MAI scores was consistent when only the non-exposed group data was analyzed, but this relationship was not significant for the cocaine exposed group data analyzed separately, suggesting a greater degree of variability in the development of the latter.

Frank and her colleagues[38] reported that the fine and gross motor movements of 6-month-old infants exposed to cocaine were rated as less optimal than unexposed infants on the Infant Behavior Record (IBR) portion of the Bayley Scales of Infant Development. They also reported a trend for lower scores on the Psychomotor Development Index scores. Statistical modeling indicated that cocaine had a direct effect on IBR motor coordination and an indirect effect through birthweight. PDI scores were also significantly related to the motor coordination scores.

Overall, findings indicate that 4-month-old infants who were exposed to cocaine in utero demonstrate delays in sensory-motor development. A significant delay remains at 12 months when an exposed group is compared to a similar group of non-exposed infants. Findings of no group difference on the Bayley Mental Scale comparisons suggest that, at 12 months of age, motor development may be a more explicit domain in which to discern developmental effects related to cocaine exposure. Failure to predict motor development in the exposed group suggests that individual subjects may demonstrate recovery or the influence of other effects during the period between 4 and 12 months.

LONG-TERM BEHAVIORAL AND COGNITIVE OUTCOMES

Given the animal literature's findings of deficits in conditioning, a basic form of learning, similar studies in human infants are of particular interest. Instrumental responses and emotional expression were assessed in a task that required infants to pull a string to elicit a visual display and musical accompaniment.[53] Infants exposed to cocaine did not master the contingency learning task as well as non-exposed infants and showed decreased arousal and lower emotional responsivity. For example, the infants exposed to cocaine failed to show frustration during the extinction phase or change in interest when the extinction phase of the experiment was discontinued.

Recent findings from one of our on-going studies[54] using 16 rating scales from the Bayley IBR indicated a significant overall group difference at 12 months of age between infants who were exposed versus non-exposed infants. Ten of the scales showed significant univariate differences. On four scales (Responsiveness to Mother, Goal Directedness, Activity, and Level of Energy), analyses suggested that a significantly greater percentage of infants exposed to cocaine fell into the suspect range. A Test Orientation and a Summary Risk score also revealed significant negative correlations with Bayley performance scores. In general, the infants appeared less socially oriented, less responsive to task and people, and less motorically coordinated than control infants. Although not matching the stereotype of hyperactivity following drug-exposure, a hesitant or inattentive child is at risk for delays.

One consistently reported association between prenatal cocaine exposure and birth outcome is intrauterine growth retardation and/or low birthweight.[55] Because low birthweight infants, especially those below 1500 grams (VLBW), are already at increased medical and developmental risk,[56] Singer and colleagues[40] investigated whether cocaine exposure was associated with greater vulnerability to neonatal medical complications or poorer developmental outcomes in very low birthweight babies. At an approximately one and a half year follow-up, 30 infants exposed to cocaine were compared to 37 control infants. Bayley Mental Development Index (MDI) and Psychomotor Development Index (PDI) scores were significantly lower in the cocaine exposed group. The authors also reported that a significantly greater percentage of the exposed infants, 33% as compared to 8% of the non-exposed infants, obtained standardized motor scores below 80. This result suggests that motor development was delayed in many of the infants exposed to cocaine. Behavioral development was also more deficient in the cocaine-exposed group, even though the VLBW comparison group was of equivalent medical risk. On a subsample rated on the IBR, cocaine exposure was related to increased bodily tension, less sustained interest in and less responsivity to test material, and less imaginative play. About one-third of the cocaine-exposed group was ranked as having "fleeting to easily distracted" attention span and as "unreactive and unresponsive."

Only one published study of long-term outcome has examined the effects of prenatal cocaine exposure on development at age 3.[8] In that report, 93 children exposed to cocaine performed more poorly than non-exposed children on the Verbal Reasoning subtest of the Stanford Binet Intelligence Scale. The majority of the children exposed to drugs, however, scored within the average range in this sample, a "best-case scenario" in which mothers received medical care and drug treatment early in their pregnancies and children were followed with intensive intervention services.

ENVIRONMENTAL CONSIDERATIONS

Our own studies in Cleveland[57] have followed a more typical cohort of infants exposed to cocaine prenatally. Identified largely at birth, the infants' mothers generally did not receive adequate prenatal care but did bring the babies for well-child care to a special interdisciplinary clinic for high-risk infants. Infants, 98% of whom were African-American and poor, were administered the Bayley Scales at 6-month intervals. The most recent follow-up included 90 cocaine-exposed and 30 non-exposed infants at mean corrected ages of 17 ± 8 months.[58] Consistent with our earlier findings, infants exposed to cocaine persisted in lagging behind the comparison group on both Mental and Motor Scale average standard scores. In this study we also assessed mothers as soon as possible after infant birth with the Brief Symptom Inventory (BSI), a standardized normative self-report of psychological symptoms (examiners were not masked as to drug status). We have found in previous work that post-partum women who were cocaine users showed an increased incidence of psychological distress, particularly paranoid ideation and phobic anxiety. When MDI scores were regressed on a summary score of the BSI and cocaine status, after controlling for infant prematurity, both variables independently predicted MDI outcome. For PDI scores, maternal psychological symptoms were not significant predictors, but the variable for cocaine use remained marginally significant ($p < .06$). These findings provide support for cocaine's direct effects on infant development and highlight the need for further studies on the effect of cocaine use on maternal psychological status because psychological status can affect maternal caregiving behavior and subsequent infant development.

METHODOLOGICAL DIFFICULTIES IN STUDYING NEUROLOGIC DEFICITS IN COCAINE-EXPOSED COHORTS

Although a growing number of published research studies and abstracts have documented a negative effect of cocaine on child neurological and developmental outcome, caution should be used when applying research findings in clinical practice. A substantial number of methodologic limitations exist in the available research literature.[59] Whether cocaine, per se, is responsible for the negative effects reported continues to be a matter of debate because the majority of samples studied have been of poor, urban women who are polydrug users. In particular, women who use cocaine tend to use alcohol, a known teratogen, more frequently than members of comparison groups, and many of the deleterious sequelae attributed to cocaine are similar to those noted in follow-up studies of fetal alcohol exposure or tobacco exposure. Scientifically, it remains important to determine cocaine's specific effects versus its confounded or synergistic effects with other substances. Pragmatically, however, infants exposed to cocaine are likely to be polydrug-exposed, and outcome or intervention studies that aim for real world validity will need to be generalizable to children as they present to clinicians.

Other methodological difficulties with the extant research literature include small sample sizes and differentially higher attrition rates in cocaine-exposed cohorts. Differential attrition may bias the sample toward those infants who are most affected and who remain in follow-up because of an identified need for service, or, alternatively, who are born at-risk and remain in follow-up because of better maternal care.

Numerous confounding factors related to maternal cocaine use continue to make it difficult to establish cocaine as a teratogen apart from associated risks of a drug-using lifestyle, including poverty, poor caretaking, poor nutrition, infections, lack of prenatal care, and premature delivery. These confounds may never be fully extricable in studies on humans.

PRACTICAL CONSIDERATIONS IN INTERVENTION

Several authors have repeated the therapeutic recommendations of Schneider[49] that delineate a programmatic effort of identification, assessment, intervention, and parent education. Identification is made most frequently on the basis of an interview. Early identification of drug exposure is difficult, however, because of the illicit nature of the drug and the mother's fear that she might go to jail and/or lose custody of her baby. Although drug screening of all pregnant women may be unfeasible and/or unwarranted, urine or, preferably, meconium testing should be considered when there is a history of inadequate prenatal care, incarceration, or previous involvement with human services agencies related to either removal of children from the home or family violence. It should be remembered that although a positive drug screen may do nothing to prevent initial drug exposure in the fetus or newborn, the information can be useful in the future when counseling the mother to quit drug use for the remainder of her current pregnancy or during future pregnancies.

When assessing infants exposed to drugs it is important not to attribute every neuromotor abnormality to cocaine. To date, many descriptions of exposure effects in infants and pre-school children are similar to those of other at-risk children. Several authors have warned against the dangers of labeling a young child.[60,61] The dangers of identifying a child as cocaine-exposed, however, should be weighed against the need for services. Unfortunately, because no specific crack-cocaine syndrome has yet been identified, labeling the "crack" baby provides no unique blueprint for intervention and may erroneously bias practitioners and educators.[62]

None of the studies published so far have suggested that standard interventions aimed at improving sensory-motor development in other at-risk infant populations would have any less success on the functioning and development of infants and young children exposed to cocaine. Consequently, therapeutic interventions commonly used to promote behavioral state regulation in children at risk as a result of prematurity, failure to thrive, or fetal alcohol exposure should be considered. Forrest[63] made several recommendations that included swaddling the infant in a semi-flexed position to reduce extensor muscle tone, using slow vertical rocking and a pacifier to prompt self-calming, and hydrotherapy. In addition, as the infant grows older, Forrest recommended avoiding placing the child in a sitting or standing position. Rather, the infant should be carried on the caregiver's hip in a flexed position facing away from the caregiver to improve trunk control and encourage reaching and grasping.

Field and her colleagues[64] reported on an intervention used with infants exposed to cocaine that was based on work with premature infants and on findings suggesting that infants exposed to cocaine display diminished performance on the response decrement items of the Brazelton Neonatal Behavioral Assessment Scale. Response decrement to repetitive external stimulation reflects the ability to shut out stimulation and is related to dopaminergic functioning in the brain. The intervention consisted of tactile-kinesthetic stimulation in the form of a slow and relatively deep pressure massage, performed in a highly specific manner. Results indicated that massage facilitated weight gain. In addition, response decrement scores approached normal.

Although a direct program of physical therapy and/or occupational therapy will not be required in most cases, Schneider[49] described several areas of parent education applicable to at-risk infants that could be applied to those exposed to cocaine. Parents can be taught to be attentive to their infant's motor behavior, noting strengths and weaknesses, and to be responsive to the individual needs of their infant. When deemed appropriate following a complete assessment, early intervention specialists should demonstrate developmentally appropriate stimulation activities and teach parents handling, range of motion, and positioning techniques that foster state regulation and normalization of muscle tone.[65]

Parent education, however, presents special challenges when adults are using drugs. Parents who use drugs may have difficulty regulating their own behavior, often relying on drugs to maintain their functioning. Parents with such problems will certainly have difficulty promoting their child's self-regulation. Attending to the infant's development and providing the appropriate activities require management of time and other resources. A drug-using lifestyle requires a person to devote much time, energy, and finances to acquiring and using the drug.[43] Without help, a parent who uses drugs may not be able to resolve the conflicting demands created by the child and the drug. The best parent education program will not benefit the child if it is not implemented. Following directions of a therapist requires compliance and acceptance of authority that is frequently absent among drug users.

CONCLUSION

The data supports the conclusion that infants exposed to cocaine in utero are at risk for delays in motor development. The extent of the risk, however, varies greatly. Developmental outcome is the product of multiple determinants, including a host of postnatal factors interacting with neurologic insults and biologic impairments. Early intervention is, therefore, both possible and often necessary. It is also important to remember that both the caregiver and the infant contribute to the developmental course. Coordinated and multifaceted efforts from numerous health care and human service disciplines are required to prevent drug exposure and, when that fails, to provide appropriate intervention.

REFERENCES

1. Frank DA, Zuckerman B, Amaro H, Aboagye K, Bauchner H, Cabral H, Fried L, Hingson R, Kayne H, Levenson SM, Parker S, Reece H, Vinci R. Cocaine use during pregnancy: Prevalence and correlates. *Pediatr.* 1988; 72:351-4.

2. Zuckerman B, Frank DA, Hingson R, Amaro H, Levenson SM, Kayne H, Parker S, Vinci R, Aboagye K, Fried LE, Cabral H, Timperi R, Bauchner H. Effects of maternal marijuana and cocaine use on fetal growth. *N Engl J Med.* 1989; 320:762-8.

3. Ostrea EM, Brady N, Gause S, Raymundo A, Stevens M. Drug screening of newborns by meconium analysis: A large-scale, prospective, epidemiologic study. *Pediatr.* 1992; 89:107-13.

4. Day NL, Cottreau CM, Richardson GA. The epidemiology of alcohol, marijuana, and cocaine use among women of childbearing age and pregnant women. *Clin Obstet Gynecol.* 1993; 36:232-245.

5. Chasnoff I, Burns K, Burns W. Cocaine use in pregnancy: Perinatal morbidity and mortality. *Neurotoxicol Teratol.* 1987; 9:291-293.

6. Chasnoff I, Burns W, Schnoll SH, Burns KA. Cocaine use in pregnancy. *N Engl J Med.* 1985; 313:666-69.

7. Chasnoff I, Chisum GM, Kaplan EW. Maternal cocaine use and genitourinary tract malformations. *Teratology.* 1988; 37:201-4.

8. Griffith D, Azuma S, Chasnoff I. Three-year outcome of children exposed prenatally to drugs. *J Am Acad Child Adolesc Psychiatry*, 1994; 33:20-7.

9. Hurt H, Brodsky NL, Betancourt L, Braitman LE, Malmud E, Giannetta J. Cocaine exposed children: Follow-up through 30 months. *Dev Behav Pediatr.* 1995; 16:29-35.

10. Woods NS, Plessinger M, Clark K. Effects of cocaine on uterine blood flow and fetal oxygenation. *JAMA*. 1987; 257:957-61.

11. Oro A, Dixon S. Perinatal cocaine and methamphetamine exposure: Maternal and neonatal correlates. *J Pediatr*. 1987; 111:571-78.

12. Schwartz KA, Cohen JA. Subarachnoid hemorrhage precipitated by cocaine snorting. *Arch Neurol*. 1984; 41:705-8.

13. Caplan LR, Hief D, Banks G. Current concepts of cerebrovascular disease-strokes and drug abuse. *Stroke*. 1982; 13: 869-72.

14. Cregler L, Mark H. Medical complications of cocaine abuse. *N Engl J Med*. 1986; 315:1499-1502.

15. Wise RA. Neural mechanisms of reinforcing action of cocaine. *National Institutes of Drug Abuse Research Monograph Series*, 1984; 50:15-23.

16. Wang C, Schnoll S. Prenatal cocaine use associated with down regulation of receptors in the human placenta. *Neurotoxicol Teratol*. 1987; 6:263-69.

17. Tennyson V, Gershon P, Budinkas M, Rothman T. Effects of extended periods of reserpine and alpha-methyl-p-tyrosine treatment on the development of putamen in fetal rabbits. *Intl J Dev Neurosci*. 1983; 1:305-18.

18. Spear L. Neurobehavioral consequences of gestational cocaine exposure: A comparative analysis. In: Rovee-Collier C, Lippsitt LP ed. *Advances in Infancy Research*, Vol 9. Norwood, NJ: Ablex; 1995;55-105.

19. Church M, Dintclieff B, Gessner P. Non-dependent consequences of cocaine on pregnancy outcome in the Long Evans rat. *Neurotoxicol Teratol*. 1988; 10:51-58.

20. Webster W, Brown-Woodman PD, Lipson A, Ritchie H. Fetal brain damage in the rat following prenatal exposure to cocaine. *Neurotoxicol Teratol*. 1991; 13:621-20.

21. Dow-Edwards DL, Freed LA, Fico TA. Structural and functional effects of prenatal cocaine exposure in adult rat brain. *Dev Brain Res*. 1990; 57:263-8.

22. Spear LP, Kirstein CL, Bell J, Yoottanasumpun V, Greenbaum R, O'Shea J, Hoffman H, Spear NE. Effects of prenatal cocaine exposure on behavior during the early postnatal period. *Neurotoxicol Teratol*. 1989; 11:57-63.

23. Heyser C, Chen W, Miller J, Spear N, Spear L. Prenatal cocaine exposure induces deficits in Pavlovian conditioning and sensory preconditioning among infant rat pups. *Behav Neurosci*. 1992; 104:955-63.

24. Riley EP, Foss JA. The acquisition of passive avoidance, active avoidance, and spatial navigation tasks by animals prenatally exposed to cocaine. *Neurotoxol Teratol*. 1991; 13:559-64.

25. Volpe J. Effects of cocaine on the fetus. *N Engl J Med*. 1992; 327:399-405.

26. Singer L, Arendt R, Song L, Warshawsky E, Kliegman R. Direct and indirect interactions of cocaine with childbirth outcomes. *Arch Pediatr Adolesc Med*. 1994; 148:959-64.

27. Frank DA, Bauchner H, Parker S, Huber AM, Kyei-Aboagye K, Cabral H, Zuckerman B. Neonatal body proportionality and body composition after in utero exposure to cocaine and marijuana. *J Pediatr*. 1990; 117:622-626.

28. Little BB, Snell LM. Brain growth among fetuses exposed to cocaine in utero. *Obstet Gynecol.* 1991; 77:361-364.

29. Dominiquez R, Vila-Coro AA, Slopis J, Bohan TP. Brain and ocular abnormalities in infants with a utero exposure to cocaine and other street drugs. *Am J Dis Child.* 1991; 145:688-95.

30. Azuma S, Chasnoff I. Outcome of children prenatally exposed to cocaine and other drugs: a path analysis of 3 year data. *Pediatr.* 1993; 92:396-402.

31. Kramer L, Locke G, Ogunyemi A, Nelson L. Neonatal cocaine related seizures. *J Child Neurol.* 1990; 5:50-64.

32. Doberczak T, Shanzer S, Senie LT, Kandall S. Neonatal neurologic and electroencephalographic effects of intrauterine cocaine exposure. *J Pediatr.* 1988; 113:354-58.

33. Legido A, Clancy R, Spitzer A, Fumegien L. Electroencephalographic and behavioral state studies in infants of cocaine-addicted mothers. *Am J Dis Child.* 1992; 146:748-52.

34. Shih L, Cone-Wesson B, Reddix B. Effects of maternal cocaine abuse on the neonatal auditory system. *Intl J Pediatr Ortholaryngol.* 1988; 15:245-51.

35. Chasnoff IJ, Bussey ME, Savic R, Stack CM. Perinatal cerebral infarction and maternal cocaine use. *J Pediatr.* 1986; 108:456-9.

36. Spires MC, Gordon EF, Chondhrire M, Maldonada E, Chan R. Intracranial hemorrhage in a neonate following prenatal cocaine exposure. *Pediatr Neurol.* 1989; 5:324-6.

37. Hoyme HE, Jones KL, Dixon SD, Jewett T, Kanson JW, Robinson LK, Msall ME, Allanson JE. Prenatal cocaine exposure and fetal vascular disruption. *Pediatr.* 1990; 85:743-7.

38. Frank DA, Jacobs RR, Park H, Cabral H, Zuckerman BS. Direct and indirect effects of cocaine exposure upon the quality of six month motor performance: Path analysis. *Pediatr Res.* 1994; 35(4) part 2:21A.

39. Dusick AM, Covert RF, Schreiber MD, Yee GT, Browne SP, Moore GM, Tebbett IR. Risk of intracranial hemorrhage and other adverse outcomes after cocaine exposure in a cohort of 323 VLBW infants. *J Pediatr.* 1993; 122:438-45.

40. Singer LT, Yamashita T, Hawkins S, Cairns D, Baley J, Kliegman R. Increased incidence of intraventricular hemorrhage and developmental delay in cocaine-exposed, very low birth weight infants. *J Pediatr.* 1994; 124:765-71.

41. Singer L, Arendt R, Minnes S. Neurodevelopmental effects of cocaine. *Clinics in Perinatology.* 1993;20(1):245-62.

42. van Baar A, de Graaff BMT. Cognitive development at preschool-age of infants of drug-dependent mothers. *Dev Med Child Neur.* 1994; 36:1063-75.

43. Howard J, Beckwith L, Rodning C, Kropenske V. The development of young children of substance-abusing parents: Insights from seven years of intervention and research. *Zero to Three.* 1989; 9:8-12.

44. Schneidner J, Chasnoff I. Motor assessment of cocaine-exposed infants. *Pediatr Res.* 1987;21:184A.

45. Dow-Edwards DL. Longterm neurochemical and neurobehavioral consequences of cocaine use during pregnancy. *Ann NY Acad Sci.* 1989; 562:280-89.

46. Bendersky M, Lewis M. Environmental risk, biological risk, and developmental outcome. *Dev Psychol.* 1994; 30:484-494.

47. Chandler LS, Andrews MS, Swanson MW. Movement Assessment of Infants: A Manual. Rolling Bay, WA: Movement Assessment of Infants; 1980.

48. Schneider JW, Lee W, Chasnoff I. Field testing of the Movement Assessment of Infants. *Phys Ther.* 1988;68:321-327.

49. Schneider JW. Motor assessment and parent education beyond the newborn period. In: Chasnoff IJ ed. *Drugs, Alcohol, Pregnancy, and Parenting.* Dordrecht: Kluwer Academic; 1988:115-125.

50. Rose-Jacobs R, Frank DA, Brown ER, Cabral H, Zuckerman BS. Use of the Movement Assessment of Infants (MAI) with in-utero cocaine-exposed infants. *Pediatr Res.* 1994; 35(4) part 2:26A.

51. Arendt R, Angelopoulos J, Bass O, Mascia, J, Singer L. Sensory-motor development in four-month-old, cocaine exposed infants. *Pediatr Res.* 1994; 35(4) part 2:18A.

52. Arendt R, Angelopoulos J, Detweiler S. Predicting Motor Development of Drug Exposed Infants. Presented at the Biennial Meeting of the Society for Research in Child Development, Indiannapolis, IN 1995.

53. Alessandri S, Sullivan M, Imaigumi S, Lewis M. Learning and emotional responsivity in cocaine exposed infants. *Dev Psych.* 1993; 6:989-97.

54. Arendt R, Angelopoulos J, Detweiller S. Behavioral patterns in cocaine exposed infants. *Pediatr Res.* 1995;37(4)part 2:248A.

55. Kliegman RM, Madura D, Kiwi R, Eisenberg I, Yamashita T. Relation of maternal cocaine use to the risks of prematurity and low birth weight. *J Pediatr.* 1994; 124:751-6.

56. Hack M, Breslau N. Biological and social determinants of 3-year IQ in very low birthweight children. In: Vietze P ed. *Early Identification of Infants with Disabilities.* New York: Grune and Stratton; 1988:41-52.

57. Singer L, Farkas K, Arendt R, Minnes S, Yamashita T, Garber R. Maternal cocaine use and psychological distress affect infant developmental outcome. *Pediatr Res.* 1995;37(4)part 2:272A.

58. Singer L, Farkas K, Arendt R, Minnes S, Yamashita T, Kliegman R. Increased psychological distress in postpartum, cocaine using mothers. *J Substance Abuse.* 1995:7:165-174.

59. Hutchings DE. The puzzle of Cocaine's effects following maternal use during pregnancy: Are there reconcilable differences? *Neurotoxicol Teratol.* 1993; 15: 281-286.

60. Coles CD. Say "Goodbye" to the "Crack Baby." *Neurotoxicol Teratol.* 1993; 15: 290-292.

61. Mayes LC, Granger RH, Bornstein MH, Zuckerman B. The problem of prenatal cocaine exposure: A rush to judgement. *Am J Obstet Gynecol.* 1987; 157:686-690.

62. Thurman KS, Brobeil RA, Ducette JP, Hurt H. Prenatally exposed to cocaine: Does the label matter? *J Early Intervention.* 1994; 18:119-130.

63. Forrest DC. The cocaine-exposed infant, part II: Intervention and teaching. *J Pediatr Health Care.* 1994; 8:7-11.

64. Wheeden A, Scafidi FA, Field T, Ironson G, Valdeon C, Bandstra E. Massage effects on cocaine-exposed preterm neonates. *Dev Behav Pediatr.* 1993; 14:318-322.

65. Huffman DL, Price BK, Langel L. Therapeutic handling techniques for the infant affected by cocaine. *Neonatal Network.* 1994; 13(5):9-13.

The Relationship Between the Movement Assessment of Infants and the Fagan Test of Infant Intelligence in Infants with Prenatal Cocaine Exposure

Dewey J. Bayer
Bruce Bleichfeld
Shelly J. Lane
Martin A. Volker
Barbara Alif
Brian Floss

SUMMARY. In the present study both the Fagan Test of Infant Intelligence (FTII) and the Motor Assessment of Infants (MAI) were administered to 36 full term infants previously exposed to cocaine *in utero*. The infants were participating in a program at the PACT (Parents And Children Together) clinic operated by Children's Hospital of Buffalo, New York. The FTII was administered at 69 weeks post-conceptional age and the MAI was administered 8 months from

Dewey J. Bayer, PhD, is Associate Professor of Psychology, and Martin A. Volker, Barbara Alif, and Brian Floss are undergraduate students, Department of Psychology, Canisius College, Buffalo, NY. Bruce Bleichfeld, PhD, is Consultant Psychologist at Children's Hospital of Buffalo, Buffalo, NY. Shelly J. Lane, PhD, OTR/L, FAOTA, is Assistant Professor, Department of Occupational Therapy, State University of New York at Buffalo, Buffalo, NY.

Address correspondence to Dewey J. Bayer, Department of Psychology, Canisius College, Buffalo, NY 14208-1098.

[Haworth co-indexing entry note]: "The Relationship Between the Movement Assessment of Infants and the Fagan Test of Infant Intelligence in Infants with Prenatal Cocaine Exposure." Bayer, Dewey J. et al. Co-published simultaneously in *Physical & Occupational Therapy in Pediatrics* (The Haworth Press, Inc.) Vol. 16, No. 1/2, 1996, pp. 145-153; and: *Children with Prenatal Drug Exposure* (ed: Lynette S. Chandler, and Shelly J. Lane) The Haworth Press, Inc., 1996, pp. 145-153. Single or multiple copies of this article are available from The Haworth Document Delivery Service [1-800-342-9678, 9:00 a.m. - 5:00 p.m. (EST). E-mail address: getinfo@haworth.com].

© 1996 by The Haworth Press, Inc. All rights reserved.

145

birth. It was hypothesized that significant relationships existed between the mean novelty preference scores on the FTII at 69 weeks and the risk scores on the subsections of the 8-month MAI. Moderate, but statistically significant, negative correlations were found between the FTII and both the automatic reactions and the primitive reflexes subsections of the MAI. The implications of these results are discussed in the context of a homeostatic model of functioning, under which the infants are viewed as having difficulties with internal regulation and motor control, leading to higher risk scores on the MAI and to lower novelty preference scores on the FTII. *[Article copies available from The Haworth Document Delivery Service: 1-800-342-9678. E-mail address: getinfo@haworth.com]*

The research literature has yielded inconsistent and often contradictory results concerning both immediate and long-term effects of *in utero* cocaine exposure,[1] and recent long-term outcome research indicates that exposed infants are not at as much risk as the literature of several years ago suggested.[2] Early effects of drug exposure are generally reported to be reflected in poor motor performance[3] and inadequate neurobehavioral functions. Motor performance abnormalities center around increased muscle tone and poorly developed primitive reflexes early in the first year, and delayed development of automatic reactions and volitional movements later in the first year. Neurobehavioral deficits noted at birth include poor state modulation and difficulty orienting and habituating to visual/auditory stimuli.[4,5] Although state modulation deficits may resolve, the outcome of poor visual orienting and habituation remains unclear.

Interestingly, one aspect of visual processing reliant on visual orientation, namely visual recognition memory (VRM), has been associated with early cognitive function. In answer to the need for early detection of later cognitive problems, the development of early infant assessment tests based on VRM has shown much promise. The tests, believed to be measures of an infant's ability to process and retain information, are based on the observation that infants tend to look longer at novel stimuli, as opposed to previously experienced stimuli, when given a choice between the two.[6,7]

The Fagan Test of Infant Intelligence (FTII) is the first standardized infant VRM test available commercially. It is utilized as a screening instrument for the early detection of infants with potential intellectual deficit.[6,7] Research has shown the FTII to be superior to traditional infant sensorimotor measures for the prediction of future cognitive outcomes.[6] It has proved to be moderately predictive of later IQ and has been shown to discriminate between control infants and infants at high risk for mental retardation or cognitive delays.[7] It is, therefore, particularly appropriate for assessing infants with prenatal substance exposure.[8]

Early assessment of motor functions can be accomplished using a variety of tools. One of these, the Movement Assessment of Infants (MAI), provides a detailed and systematic means of evaluating motor behaviors in infants.[9,10] It is both a quantitative and a qualitative measure used to evaluate muscle tone, primitive reflexes, automatic reactions, and volitional movements.[9,10,11]

According to Greenspan and Lourie,[12] the most important initial task of an infant is to achieve homeostasis. This capacity, which normally develops over the first three months after birth, consists of the infant being able to adapt or attend to the external environment and simultaneously maintain a state of internal regulation.[12] Such skill requires the interaction of many systems. We suggest that motor system function provides a physical foundation upon which visual orientation and attention and behavioral regulation are imposed in the production of homeostasis. Problems in homeostatic functioning are therefore thought to be reflected in higher risk scores on the MAI, as well as in difficulties with attention resulting in lower mean novelty preference scores on the FTII.

Recent studies would seem to support this expectation in demonstrating both elevated MAI risk scores in full term cocaine/polydrug-exposed infants at four months of age,[3,13] and difficulties with alertness, state control, and attention in exposed infants during the first four months of life and later into the first year.[14] Struthers and Hansen[14] also reported that mean novelty preference scores on the FTII, given between 69 and 92 weeks post-conceptional age, were significantly lower for infants exposed to stimulant drugs (predominantly cocaine) *in utero* than for controls.

Thus, previous research has determined that homeostatic disturbance occurs as a result of cocaine exposure *in utero*, and we suggest that this may be a function of both motor and neurobehavioral deficits. As such, this study was carried out to examine the potential relationship between motor performance and VRM using the four MAI sections and the mean novelty preference score of the FTII, in a group of infants exposed to cocaine and tested near 8 months of age.

METHOD

Subjects

The sample was comprised of 36 fullterm infants (37 to 41 weeks post-conceptional age at birth) born at Children's Hospital in Buffalo, New York, between February 1990 and July 1992. The 20 females and 16 males were identified as prenatally exposed to cocaine either by testing positive for the cocaine metabolite benzoylecgonine in a urine toxicology screening, or on the basis of the mother's admission to using cocaine during the pregnancy. All of the mothers were receiving social welfare support (Medicaid), and the sample's racial composition consisted of 33 African-American infants, 2 Hispanic, and 1 Caucasian infant. Most (25) of the mothers had received prenatal care; 17 of the infants had been placed in foster care shortly after birth. The sample was drawn from a larger cohort of over 400 children identified as cocaine-exposed and receiving primary care in the Hospital's PACT (Parents And Children Together) Clinic. PACT was developed under federal Maternal and Child Health funding to give medical care and social support to infants who were substance-exposed and their families.

Instrumentation

The Movement Assessment of Infants (MAI) consists of a total of 65 items distributed over four sections–Muscle Tone, Primitive Reflexes, Automatic Reactions, and Volitional Movement.[9] An a priori profile of expected infant performance, at both 4 and 8 months of age, is provided for comparative purposes.[9,17] The MAI is scored by the accumulation of risk points. One risk point is assigned for each item on which the infant deviates from expected performance. Risk points are then totaled for each subsection and for the test as a whole. A total of 48 risk points can be accumulated on the 4-month profile, and a total of 61 risk points on the 8-month profile. The increased risk point potential at 8 months reflects an increase in performance expectations in the automatic reaction and volitional movement sections of the MAI. The MAI can be administered by an experienced evaluator in 20-30 minutes.

The Fagan Test of Infant Intelligence (FTII) is a standardized test of visual recognition memory (VRM).[6,7] The test consists of 10 novelty problems, made up of achromatic and colored pictures of human faces, given to infants at 67, 69, 79, and/or 92 weeks post-conceptional age. Each novelty problem consists of showing the infant one picture (or, at times, two pictures) of a human face for a standard time and then pairing that picture with a new, novel picture for a standard time. The tester records the length of time the infant spends looking at each picture by watching corneal reflections through a magnified peephole in the test screen. A novelty preference score is then calculated by dividing the amount of time the infant spends looking at the novel picture by the total amount of time spent looking at both pictures, multiplied by 100. A mean novelty preference score is then determined by averaging the scores for all 10 novelty problems. Infants with scores ≤ 53 are considered to be at risk. The FTII can be administered by an experienced tester in 20-25 minutes.

Procedure

The infants were tested on the FTII and MAI on separate occasions. The MAI was administered at 8 months ± 2 weeks chronologic age during regularly scheduled appointments at the PACT Clinic. The FTII was administered at 69 weeks ± 1 week post-conceptional age at the Neuro-behavioral Clinic of Buffalo General Hospital. Because the FTII was administered at a different location and was unrelated to regularly scheduled PACT Clinic appointments, a greater degree of self-selection was expected for FTII subjects, and, indeed, many subjects failed to show up for their FTII appointments. This resulted in only 50% of the total number of subjects referred for FTII testing actually being tested.

RESULTS

The data collected and analyzed were, for the MAI, the total risk points on each of the four sections (Muscle Tone, Primitive Reflexes, Automatic Reactions, and Volitional Movements) and, for the FTII, the mean novelty preference scores. Summary statistics can be found in Table 1. Correlation coefficients were computed among these five measures, and the resulting correlation matrix can be found in Table 2. Significant negative relationships were found between the FTII and both Automatic Reactions ($r = -.32$, $p < .05$) and Primitive Reflexes ($r = -.33$, $p < .05$) Risk Scores. Also significant, though not relevant to the hypothesis being tested, were several of the correlations among the MAI sub-sections Risk Scores.

TABLE 1. Means and Standard Deviations of Risk Scores for the MAI Subsections at 8 Months and the FTII Mean Novelty Preference Scores at 69 Weeks

Test	N	Mean	Std Dev	Range
Primitive Reflexes	36	1.06	1.17	0-4
Automatic Reactions	36	2.06	2.07	0-10
Muscle Tone	36	2.53	2.30	0-7
Volitional Movement	36	2.56	3.26	0-13
FTII Mean 69 Weeks	36	62.83	7.28	44-75.6

TABLE 2. Intercorrelations Between FTII at 69 Weeks and MAI Sub-Sections at 8 Months

Test/Section	Automatic Reactions	Muscle Tone	Volitional Movement	Primitive Reflexes
	Cocaine-exposed infants ($\underline{n}$ = 36)			
FTII	−.3269*	−.0162	−.1924	−.3329*
Automatic Reactions	−	.4141*	.4576**	.3292*
Muscle Tone		−	.3491*	.4457**
Volitional Movement			−	−.0008
Primitive Reflexes				−

*$p < .05.$ **$p < .01.$

On the FTII, the average mean novelty preference score for the 36 infants was 62.83, with a range of 44.0 to 75.6. Only 4 of the 36 subjects fell into the at-risk range (mean novelty preference score ≤ 53).

DISCUSSION

Our findings indicate that for infants exposed prenatally to cocaine there is a significant relationship between some aspects of motor development, as assessed by the MAI, and visual recognition memory, as assessed by the FTII. Specifically, as the number of motor problems increase (as indicated by MAI risk points on Automatic Reactions and on Primitive Reflexes), mean novelty preference scores on the FTII decrease. Novelty preference is viewed as an early predictor of later cognitive growth, and the relationship found in the present study has implications for the importance of the integration of early motor and attentional processes for later cognitive development.

Only two of the four MAI sections, Automatic Reactions and Primitive Reflexes, were significantly correlated with the FTII. The Automatic Reactions section assesses head righting reactions, equilibrium responses, and protective extension responses. The Primitive Reflexes section measures the asymmetrical tonic neck reflex, both spontaneous and evoked; the palmar and plantar grasp reflexes; the tonic labyrinthine reflexes in prone and supine; the positive support reflex; the walking reflex; the Moro reflex; and the Galant reflex. Thus, both of these sections address motor skills important to the infant's ability to maintain a stable sitting position when perturbed, and to dissociate head and trunk movements. These motor abilities provide a foundation for the expression of cognitive function in the infant. When these motor skills are poorly developed, i.e., when MAI risk points in these sections are high, the infant may find it difficult to express cognitive functions such as VRM because attention is directed toward maintaining the upright posture and imposing movement of the head on trunk stability. Thus, these findings support a possible linkage between motor and attentional integration in infancy and cognitive development, a linkage which has been implied in the Developmental Structuralist model of Greenspan.[12,15,16] According to the model, an infant must modulate multisensory inputs while maintaining a calm affective state. The infant's ability to perform this modulation corresponds to its capacity to achieve homeostasis or self-regulation. A child who must struggle to control motor adjustments would not be able to attend visually in an adaptive way.

A recent study by Struthers and Hansen[14] found that infants who were prenatally drug-exposed scored lower on the FTII than non-exposed infants, leading to concern over early cognitive performance. It is noteworthy, however, that the drug-exposed infants in the Struthers and Hansen study received an average score of 58.9, clearly above the cut-off suggested by Fagan as indicative of problems with VRM. The mean score of the infants in our study (62.8) slightly exceeded this value. This difference may be attributable to our use of only the 69-week FTII values, while Struthers and Hansen obtained mean values from both the 69- and 92-week assessment times. The FTII is known to have low consistency from one testing to another,[6,7] and it may be that if they had only tested at 69 weeks, they would have obtained scores similar to ours. The subjects in the present study were also participants in a clinic intervention program from birth. They received a wealth of social support from birth through the assessment period and this may have had a positive influence on FTII performance.

The findings in the present study support our contention that motor system function provides a physical foundation upon which visual orientation and attention and behavioral regulation are imposed in the production of homeostasis. This statement of relationship, however, is tempered by the recognition that the study's design does not allow cause/effect conclusions. In fact, the MAI assessment took place about 1-2 months later than the FTII assessment. Those who came for the FTII assessment were a self-selected group, which may also contribute to a non-representative finding. Similar confirming research must be done with more representative samples and with both normal infants and infants at risk for reasons other than prenatal drug exposure. A need also exists for more research on both visual recognition memory and its importance in the development of the infant. Also, increased attempts must be made to differentiate between the teratogenic effects of substances and both constitutional characteristics of the child and environmental factors associated with drug-using homes.

ACKNOWLEDGMENTS

We would like to extend our thanks to the participating families, all PACT clinic staff, and graduate students who participated in data collection. In addition, we would like to thank Dr. David Shucard, Director of the Neurobehavioral Sciences Laboratory at Buffalo General Hospital for the use of the Fagan test materials.

REFERENCES

1. Myers BJ, Olson HC, Kaltenbach K. Cocaine-exposed infants: Myths and misunderstandings. *Zero To Three.* 1992;13(1):1-5.

2. Griffith, D, Azuma, S, Chasnoff, I. Three-year outcome of children exposed prenatally to drugs. *J Am Aca Child Adol Psychiatr.* 1993;33(1), 20-27.

3. Schneider JW, Griffith DR, Chasnoff IJ. Infants exposed to cocaine in utero: Implications for developmental assessment and intervention. *Inf Young Child.* 1989;2(1):25-36.

4. Chasnoff IJ, Lewis DE, Griffith DR, Willey S. Cocaine and pregnancy: Clinical and toxicology implications for the neonate. *Clini Chem.* 1989;35:1276-1278.

5. Hadeed AJ, Siegel SR. Maternal cocaine use during pregnancy: Effect on the newborn infant. *Pediatr.* 1989;84:205-210.

6. Benasich, AA, Bejar, II. The Fagan Test of Infant Intelligence: A critical view. *J App Dev Psychol.* 1992;13:153-171.

7. Fagan JF, Detterman DK. The Fagan Test of Infant Intelligence: A technical summary. *J Appl Dev Psychol.* 1992;13:173-193.

8. Scott KG, Urbano JC, Boussy CA. Long-term psychoeducational outcome of prenatal substance exposure. *Sem Perinat.* 1991;15(4):317-323.

9. Chandler, LS, Andrews MS, Swanson MW. *Movement Assessment of Infants: A Manual.* Rolling Bay, WA: Authors; 1980.

10. Harris SR, Haley SM, Tada WL, Swanson MW. Reliability of observational measures of the Movement Assessment of Infants. *Phys Ther.* 1984;64:471-477.

11. Haley SM, Harris SR, Tada WL, Swanson MW. Item reliability of the Movement Assessment of Infants. *Phys Occupa Ther Ped.* 1986;6(1):21-39.

12. Greenspan S, Lourie RS. Developmental structuralist approach to the classification of adaptive and pathologic personality organizations: Infancy and early childhood. *Am J Psychiatr.* 1981;138(6):725-735.

13. Schneider JW, Chasnoff IJ. Motor assessment of cocaine/polydrug exposed infants at age 4 months. *Neurotoxicol Teratol*. 1992;14(2):91-101.

14. Struther JM, Hansen RL. Visual recognition memory in drug-exposed infants. *J Dev Behav Ped*. 1992;13(2):108-111.

15. Greenspan S. Regulatory disorders I: Clinical perspectives. *NIDA Res Mono*. 1991;114:165-172.

16. Greenspan S. *Infancy and Early Childhood*. Madison, CT: International Universities Press; 1992.

17. Chandler LS, Andrews MS, Swanson MW, Larson EB. *Scoring Sheet for Movement Assessment of Infants with Eight-month Profile*. Rolling Bay, WA: Authors; 1988.

Development of Children in Foster Care: Comparison of Battelle Screening Test Performance of Children Prenatally Exposed to Cocaine and Non-Exposed Children

Laura M. Giusti

SUMMARY. Twenty-four foster children aged 12 to 28 months were assessed using the Battelle Developmental Inventory Screening Test (BDI).[1] A subset of the children (15) had been exposed to cocaine in utero. All of the children were of African-American descent; eight of the drug-exposed and five of the non-exposed children were female. Results of t-tests for total and domain scores on the BDI suggested that there were no significant developmental differences between the drug-exposed and non-exposed groups. Overall, however, the sample of foster children scored lower than average on the national norms for the BDI, and their age equivalents as measured by the BDI were significantly lower than their actual ages.

Laura M. Giusti, MA, is completing an internship at the Brown Consortium in Clinical Child Psychology and will have her PhD in Child Psychology conferred by the University of Kansas in 1996. She initiates postdoctoral studies at the Emma P. Bradley Hospital, at Brown University, Providence, RI in July 1996 in Clinical Child Psychology.
This study was supported in part by a Research Fellowship from the University of Kansas Graduate School. Permission for this study was granted by Judge Michael Coburn of the Circuit Court of Jackson County, MO.

[Haworth co-indexing entry note]: "Development of Children in Foster Care: Comparison of Battelle Screening Test Performance of Children Prenatally Exposed to Cocaine and Non-Exposed Children." Giusti, Laura M. Co-published simultaneously in *Physical & Occupational Therapy in Pediatrics* (The Haworth Press, Inc.) Vol. 16, No. 1/2, 1996, pp. 155-171; and: *Children with Prenatal Drug Exposure* (ed: Lynette S. Chandler, and Shelly J. Lane) The Haworth Press, Inc., 1996, pp. 155-171. Single or multiple copies of this article are available from The Haworth Document Delivery Service [1-800-342-9678, 9:00 a.m. - 5:00 p.m. (EST). E-mail address: getinfo@haworth.com].

© 1996 by The Haworth Press, Inc. All rights reserved.

Possible explanations are discussed, including the diminution of adverse effects of prenatal cocaine-exposure, as well as the overall poor developmental outcome of foster children. *[Article copies available from The Haworth Document Delivery Service: 1-800-342-9678. E-mail address: getinfo@haworth.com]*

On any given day, there are an estimated three to four hundred thousand children in foster care in the United States.[2] Most of these children are placed in foster homes because they have been abused or neglected by their parents. In addition to their abusive or neglectful environments, most of the children that enter foster care come from families struggling with poverty and cultural deprivation.[2-4] Frequent changes in foster home placement, changes in the other members present in the foster home, uncertain length of placement, and discontinued or infrequent contact with their biologic parents are potential obstacles to the children's healthy psychological and emotional development.[3,5-6] For these reasons, foster care is a less than ideal placement for children who have already been stressed by their families of origin. More recently, additional discouraging evidence about the status of children in foster care has emerged.

Recent studies suggest that children in foster care are in poor physical and emotional health.[2-4,7-8] Because of the very reasons they entered the foster care system, these children are in need of special care for physical or emotional problems and risks. Further evidence suggests that children in foster care do not receive the medical assistance necessary to effectively manage these problems.[2,4,9]

The mental health of children in foster care appears to be compromised in a variety of domains. In their reviews, Klee and Halfon[10] and Hochstadt and colleagues[2] found that many large studies report a variety of cognitive, behavioral, psychosocial and developmental problems among children in foster care. McIntyre and Keesler[3] concluded that previous studies have documented the high frequency of psychologic disorders among foster children in general. The majority of these studies, however, are based on assessments conducted with older children. Little data exists concerning the mental health status of young children in foster care. The effects of abuse and neglect, as well as foster care placement, may be manifested differentially according to the developmental stage of the child in care.[11] It is important, therefore, that the mental health status of infants and toddlers be assessed with age-appropriate instruments.

One special subset of these young children in foster care is the increasing number who have been placed because of suspected or confirmed prenatal maternal drug use. In the past five years, more women appear to be using cocaine during pregnancy and with more frequency than other illicit drugs.[12] It is estimated that between 10-20% of newborns in urban nurseries and intensive care units have been affected by maternal prenatal cocaine use.[13-14] Prenatal use of cocaine has been reported to have adverse effects on the developing fetus and neonate.[12,15-18] Cocaine-associated neonatal complications include congenital malformations, decreased fetal growth, preterm delivery, seizures, cerebral infarctions, sudden infant death syndrome, cardiac arrhythmias, and behavioral changes.[19] Very little has been reported on the effects of cocaine exposure after infancy.[20] Emerging evidence suggests that many of the initial adverse outcomes, such as low birth weight, small stature, and preterm delivery, do not continue to pose problems as the child develops.[20] At least one study suggests that the adverse neurologic effects of cocaine exposure decrease after infancy.[21]

The majority of studies that have reported adverse outcomes of prenatal exposure to cocaine in neonates were focused almost exclusively on the infants' motor, perceptual, and neurobehavioral functions.[20] Assessment of an infant's mental health has rarely been included in such studies. In addition, very few studies have conducted follow-up assessments with prenatally exposed children to determine the longer term effects on emotional and psychologic development. The majority of the mental health studies that have been conducted have used the Neonatal Behavioral Assessment Scale (NBAS),[22] which is designed for use only during the first month of life. Singer and colleagues[12] reported that, with the exception of one study, the NBAS results revealed sensory and behavioral deficits in infants exposed to cocaine in comparison to non-cocaine-exposed controls. They also reported that the pattern of abnormalities is inconsistent and that further studies with larger samples and better control groups are warranted.[12] Finally, Singer and associates[12] reported equivocal results from studies that had investigated toddler development and could only conclude that cocaine-exposure leads to risk for later learning and behavioral disabilities.

Increasing evidence suggests that the care-taking environment of children who were drug-exposed may be as influential on later development as the drug exposure itself. In their study of poly-drug users and their newborns, Chasnoff and colleagues[20] reported that at two-year follow-up development was comparable to that of drug-free infants. They added that both the drug-exposed and non-exposed groups were demonstrating a downward trend in developmental scores which is not uncommon in infants from low socioeconomic milieus.[20] In fact, Chasnoff, Schnoll, Burns, and Burns[23] and Kaltenbach and Finnegan[24] have argued that environmental factors such as low socioeconomic status, poor housing, and stress have been shown to have as much of an effect on developmental outcomes as has prenatal drug exposure. These environmental factors are also associated with child abuse and neglect and therefore are likely to have been experienced by children who enter foster care. In order to effectively intervene with both drug-exposed and non-exposed children who demonstrate psychosocial and developmental deficiencies, it is essential that we understand the nature of their problem. To create effective treatment and prevention strategies we must determine the differential impact of drug-exposure versus the drug-use environment. Additional research is needed to discriminate among these effects.

In summary, in the cases of infant and toddler children in foster care, and toddlers exposed to cocaine, further studies of development are needed to investigate their mental health and developmental status, and to begin to distinguish the effects of drug-exposure from the effects of an associated impoverished environment. In the present study, 24 children aged 12 to 28 months and in foster care, 15 of whom had been prenatally exposed to cocaine, were assessed using the Battelle Developmental Inventory Screening test (BDI).[1] The study questions were as follows:

1. Do toddlers in foster care who were drug-exposed perform below standardized norms on the BDI?
2. Do toddlers in foster care who were not drug-exposed perform below standardized norms on the BDI?
3. Do toddlers in foster care who were drug-exposed score lower on average than non-exposed toddlers on the BDI?

METHOD

Subjects

Subjects included 24 toddlers in the Jackson County, Missouri, foster care system. Only African-American subjects were included because of the small number of Caucasian infants identified as drug-exposed in this county. After permission for the study was granted by the county and state, the Missouri Division of Family Services (DFS) produced a list of all African-American toddlers aged 12 to 36 months currently in foster care who were identified as cocaine-exposed by toxicology screen or maternal report at the time of birth. An additional group of African-American toddlers in foster care were identified as non-exposed. The non-exposed group consisted of toddlers whose mothers did not report drug use during their pregnancies, and either were not subjected to toxicology screens, or received negative toxicology screens after their child's delivery. The researchers were given the toddlers' foster names, addresses, and phone numbers, but were not informed of the toddlers' drug exposure status. Of the original 38 foster mothers who were contacted, 9 chose not to participate, most citing time constraints. No information was available about the children of those foster mothers who chose not to participate. Of the 29 foster mothers who agreed to participate, Battelle data were analyzed for 24 of the children. Of the five subjects excluded, two were dropped because the status of their drug-exposure was unclear, one was dropped because he was diagnosed as having cerebral palsy, one was dropped because she was Caucasian, and one was dropped because of experimenter error.

Of the 24 subjects, 15 were identified as cocaine-exposed, and 9 as not having been exposed to illicit drugs prenatally. Drug exposure was defined as the prenatal use of cocaine only, or of cocaine in combination with alcohol, marijuana, or cigarettes (see Tables 1 and 2 for additional information about the subjects).

TABLE 1. Prenatal Drug Exposure

Subject Number	Cocaine	Alcohol	Marijuana	Nicotine
222	X	X	X	X
261	X	X	X	X
152	X	X	X	?
13	X	X		X
189	X	X		X
306	X	X		X
164	X	X		X
66	X		X	X
221	X	X		
257	X	X		
193	X			X
47	X		X	
91	X			X
16	X			?
158	X			?

TABLE 2. Age in Months and Length of Time in Placement

Subject Number	Gender	Age in Months	Time in Placement
Cocaine-Exposed			
261	F	12	12
16	M	14	14
47	F	15	1
152	M	18	16
164	M	20	19
189	M	20	20
66	F	21	21
91	F	22	22
158	F	22	22
193	M	23	22
13	F	24	?
222	F	24	24
221	F	25	24
306	M	27	27
257	M	28	12
Non-Exposed			
200	F	12	7
155	M	15	15
301	F	16	12
128	M	18	18
114	F	19	8
266	M	22	6
56	M	23	10
55	F	23	10
302	F	27	12

Powder cocaine use and crack cocaine use were not differentiated through toxicology screen of maternal report. Subjects in the control group were placed in foster care because of parental child abuse or neglect. Because of DFS's concerns about maintaining their clients' confidentiality, and the lack of complete records, additional information about the toddlers' birth weight, gestational age, and the course of prenatal care was unavailable for most of the toddlers.

Measures

Demographic Survey. Demographic information, including the age and gender of the toddler; the foster mother's age, education, and income; and the length of time the child had been in foster care placement, was collected through an interview with the foster parent.

The Battelle Developmental Inventory Screening Test. The Battelle Developmental Inventory[1] is a standardized instrument used to assess developmental skills in children from birth to 8 years. The full inventory consists of 341 items distributed across five developmental domains including Personal-Social, Adaptive, Motor, Communication, and Cognitive. The Battelle Developmental Inventory Screening Test includes a subject of 96 items from the five domains of the full inventory. In the Screening Test each item is presented in a standardized format and scored with a three-point scoring system which takes into account developing as well as achieved skills.

Each of the domains assesses different types of skills. The 20 Personal-Social domain items assess the child's ability to engage in meaningful social interactions. Examples of items for infants and toddlers include, "Shows awareness of his/her hands," "Plays peekaboo," and "Imitates another child or children at play." The 20 Adaptive domain items measure the child's ability to make use of information and accomplish self-help and task-related skills. Examples include, "Takes strained food from spoon and swallows," "Removes small articles of clothing without assistance," and "Distinguishes between food substances and nonfood substances." The 20 Motor domain items assess the child's ability to initiate an activity, to remain on task, and to receive satisfaction from achievements. Item examples include, "Moves object in hand to mouth," "Moves three or more feet by crawling," and "Places four rings on post in any order." In the motor domain, both gross and fine motor skills are assessed and can be scored independently as sub-domain scores. The 18 Communication domain items assess the child's reception and expression of information, thoughts and ideas. Examples of the domain items include, "Turns head toward source of sound outside field of vision," "Associates spoken words with familiar objects or actions," and "Uses ten or more words." Receptive and expressive communication can also be scored independently as sub-domain scores. The 18 items from the Cognitive domain measure skills that are conceptual in nature and are related to perceptual discrimination, memory, and reasoning skills. Examples of items include "Follows visual stimulus," "Searches for removed object," and "Recognizes self as cause of events or happenings." During test administration, the examiner uses a standard set of objects and inquiries to elicit behaviors and skills from the child. Those items that cannot or have not been clearly assessed and scored through direct observation or interaction are scored using caretaker reports of the child's behaviors.

Preliminary studies suggest that the concurrent and criterion-related validity of the Battelle Developmental Inventory are good,[25-26] but similar studies on the 96 subset of items that comprise the Battelle Developmental Inventory Screening Test have not yet been conducted. The internal consistency and test-retest reliability coefficients for the Screening Test are high.[1] The normative data for the Screening Test were collected on 800 children from all regions of the country at ages from birth to 95 months. The sample included 16% minority children and 50% females, reflecting the national population distributions.

Procedure

The Missouri DFS located the names, addresses, and phone numbers of foster parents and their children who met our inclusionary criteria and contacted them by letter to inform them of our study. DFS then gave the names and phone numbers to the investigators who contacted the eligible subjects by phone to solicit their participation. If the foster parents agreed to participate after being informed about the study, a home interview was scheduled.

A graduate student researcher and an undergraduate research assistant served as administrators of the BDI assessment. Both were trained by use of the BDI manual, videotaped practice, and the testing of pilot subjects. Both assessors were unaware of the drug status of the subjects during testing. The toddlers were assessed in their foster home with the foster parent present but not in the same room. The BDI was administered after 5-10 minutes of establishing rapport with the child and took approximately twenty minutes to administer.

RESULTS

Description of the Sample

The subjects ranged in age from 12 to 28 months, with a mean age in the cocaine-exposed group of 21.0, and a mean age in the non-exposed group of 19.4. There was no significant difference between groups on age $\{t(1) = .624, p > .05\}$. The cocaine-exposed and non-exposed groups did not differ significantly on the income, education, marital status, or age of the foster mother, but there was a significant difference between groups on length of time in placement. Toddlers in the drug-exposed group had been in placement significantly longer (mean = 19.3 months) than non-exposed toddlers (mean = 10.9 months) at the time of testing (Tables 2 and 3).

The Battelle Developmental Inventory

To score the Battelle, all item scores are summed to create sub-domain and domain total scores in the Personal-Social, Adaptive, Motor, Communication, and Cognitive skills categories. The domain totals are then summed to create the total score. Subjects' sub-domain, domain, and total score are compared with the Battelle standardized norms and determined to be comparable to the norm or as 1, 1.5, or 2 standard deviations (SD) below the norm. In addition, each subject's raw score for the sub-domains, domains, and total score were compared with normed data and given an age-equivalent score.

A t-test was conducted between group means on the total raw score including all items. An additional t-test was conducted between groups on the subsequently derived age-equivalent scores. There were no significant differences across group or sex for total raw scores or age-equivalent scores (Tables 4 and 5). Even though the overall score totals did not differ significantly between groups, for the sake of completeness t-tests were also conducted between group means on sub-domain raw scores. There were no significant differences across group or sex for the sub-domain scores (Tables 4 and 5).

Because no statistically significant differences were detected between the drug-exposed and non-exposed groups, the samples were collapsed for additional analyses. Each individual subject's Battelle raw score was compared against their age-appropriate norm and then classified as falling above or below the norm for Chi square analysis. Although the Chi square analysis was non-significant ($X^2 = 1.60, p = .20$), 15 of the 24 subjects fell

TABLE 3. Means, Standard Deviations, and t Values for Age in Months and Length of Time in Placement by Group

	Cocaine-Exposed n = 15		Non-Exposed n = 9		Test of Significance
Age in Months	M =	19.4	M =	21.0	
	SD =	4.72	SD =	4.64	t (22) = .624
Length of Time in Placement	M =	19.29	M =	10.89	
	SD =	4.75	SD =	3.85	t (22) = 19.70*

*p < .001.

TABLE 4. Means, Standard Deviations, and t Values for Battelle Raw Scores by Group

Domain	Cocaine-Exposed n = 15		Non-Exposed n = 9		Test of Significance
Personal Social	M = 13.53	SD = 4.31	M = 13.56	SD = 3.17	t = .0002
Adaptive	M = 13.67	SD = 3.15	M = 14.11	SD = 3.44	t = .1044
Motor	M = 13.00	SD = 4.04	M = 13.67	SD = 2.4	t = .2007
Communication	M = 12.07	SD = 4.77	M = 11.33	SD = 2.35	t = .1834
Cognitive	M = 10.60	SD = 2.72	M = 10.67	SD = 1.50	t = .0045
TOTAL SCORE	M = 63.53	SD = 15.15	M = 63.33	SD = 11.73	t = .0011

below their standardized norm (Table 6). In addition, a paired t-test found that children's age equivalents (mean = 16.21, SD = 5.06) as scored by the Battelle, were significantly lower than their actual ages (mean = 20.42, SD = 4.63; $t(23) = 6.02$, $p < .0001$) (Table 7).

DISCUSSION

In response to the original study questions, the results of this study suggest that there were no differences on the BDI between toddlers in foster care who were or were not cocaine-exposed. The results also suggest, however, that as a whole the foster children scored below the BDI norm group and below their chronologic age expectations on the BDI. There are many possible explanations for these results.

First, the lack of differences between children who were or were not drug-exposed may be related to the many sociocultural variables that influence children's health and development. It is likely that all foster children, including those placed because of prenatal exposure to drugs as well as those placed because of abuse or neglect, demonstrate some developmental delays or difficulties based on environmental influences. Adult

TABLE 5. Means, Standard Deviations, and t Values for Battelle Raw Scores by Sex

Domain	Male (n = 11)		Female (n = 13)		Test of Significance
Personal Social	M =	15.09	M =	12.23	t = 3.6822
	SD =	.09	SD =	3.22	
Adaptive	M =	14.27	M =	13.46	t = .3727
	SD =	3.41	SD =	3.10	
Motor	M =	13.91	M =	12.69	t = .7250
	SD =	2.98	SD =	3.86	
Communication	M =	12.73	M =	11.00	t = 1.1232
	SD =	2.95	SD =	2.20	
Cognitive	M =	11.09	M =	10.23	t = .8274
	SD =	2.95	SD =	1.59	
TOTAL SCORE	M =	67.09	M =	60.38	t = 1.4571
	SD =	16.90	SD =	9.96	

TABLE 6. Cocaine-Exposed and Non-Exposed Toddlers' Scores Above or Below Norm for Age

	Drug-Exposed	Non-Exposed	Total
Below Norm	10	5	15
At or Above Norm	5	4	9
Total	15	9	

TABLE 7. Comparison of Age in Months and Age Equivalents by Subject

Subject	Age in Months	Age Equivalents
Cocaine-Exposed		
261	12	12
16	14	8
47	15	12
152	18	15
164	20	12
189	20	16
66	21	15
91	22	15
158	22	20
193	23	18
222	24	14
13	24	15
221	25	17
306	27	25
257	28	30
Non-Exposed		
200	12	10
155	15	16
301	16	8
128	18	14
114	19	21
266	22	20
55	23	17
56	23	19
302	27	20

$$M = 20.4167 \qquad M = 16.2083$$
$$SD = 4.634 \qquad SD = 5.056$$

$$t (23) = 6.02****$$

****$p < .0001$

drug use is associated with low socioeconomic status, poor nutrition, lack of prenatal care, and family instability, factors which can adversely affect fetal and child development. Singer and colleagues[12] suggest the "Maternal and environmental correlates of crack-cocaine use, such as poverty, domestic violence, foster care, and neglect, also negatively affect cognitive and emotional competence in the over 100,000 infants born annually with exposure to cocaine" (p.403). Others suggest that environmental factors such as low socioeconomic status, poor housing, and stress have been shown to have as much of an effect on developmental outcomes as prenatal drug exposure.[23-24] Although prenatal exposure to cocaine may cause early, adverse physiologic effects, it is likely that they diminish over time[20] and remaining signs and symptoms may be more closely associated with the adverse sociocultural conditions. Similarly, child abuse and neglect are associated with lower sociocultural status and stress.[27-29] Abuse and neglected children are at risk for many of the same adverse effects of impoverished and chaotic environments as are children who are drug-exposed. This similarity of environmental adversity is one possible explanation for the lack of differences between the cocaine-exposed and non-exposed toddlers' developmental scores, and their uniformly low scores in their sample. Whereas their drug-exposure history differs, both the toddlers who were drug-exposed and the non-exposed toddlers probably experienced adverse prenatal and early environmental conditions that influenced their development.

We conclude that the toddlers' pre- and postnatal environmental adversities may have affected their development more than did the cocaine exposure. Because this sample of drug-exposed children did not return to, or remain in, their biologic home with their drug-abusing parent for more than a month in almost all cases, one could conclude that it was the drug-abusing mother's environment and lifestyle during her *pregnancy* that affected the fetus' health and development, and which continued to affect the developing child. However, because of the stresses associated with foster care, we cannot assume that all foster care experiences and environments promote appropriate child development. Therefore, it is possible that these foster care system stresses may have exacerbated the toddlers' existing predisposition to low scores on the BDI, or contributed solely to the low scores. Further research is needed to isolate and measure the effects of specific stressors in the foster care system.

Another possible explanation for the lack of differences between the cocaine-exposed and non-exposed groups is that the Battelle Screening test was insensitive to the relevant differences. Although there has been some preliminary support for the Battelle Developmental Inventory's concurrent validity, interrater, and test-retest reliability,[25] little has been reported for the Screening test. It is possible that the larger battery would have detected differences that the Screening test was not able to because the Screening test assesses a smaller range of skills.

On another aspect of the issue of test appropriateness, Chasnoff and colleagues[20] suggest that standard developmental tests may not capture the deficits caused by prenatal exposure to cocaine. They cite anecdotal reports suggesting that some cocaine-exposed children have low thresholds for overstimulation and difficulties with self-regulation, deficits which are rarely assessed in existing developmental tests and dimensions which are not assessed in the BDI. It is possible that the deficits of children exposed to cocaine (and their differences from non-exposed children) will become more apparent as we design instruments that are capable of assessing the relevant symptoms.

Furthermore, the lack of differences between the drug-exposed and non-exposed groups at this point in their development does not rule out the possibility that the toddlers exposed to drugs will experience adverse effects later in their development. "Sleeper effects" of the drug exposure may become evident in the form of developmental or other problems.[20]

Finally, the lack of differences between the cocaine-exposed and non-exposed toddlers' scores could be the result of methodologic problems in the study. The first possible problem that may account for the lack of significant differences was that we were unable to unequivocally confirm that some drug-exposed toddlers had not mistakenly been placed in the non-exposed group. It is unknown whether the mothers of the children in the control group were ever tested for drug-use during their pregnancy. The mistaken placement of some drug-exposed children in the non-exposed group may have contributed to the lack of differences and overall low scores in the sample. Future studies should attempt to conduct regular toxicology screens throughout the duration of the women's pregnancy to insure accurate group assignment.

Second, the lack of differences could be explained by the low statistical power to detect differences caused by the small number of subjects available for testing. The small number of subjects is a common problem in conducting research with this type of population.[12] Until longitudinal studies are available, accumulating information from many small studies will be both necessary and valuable in our attempts to understand the long-term effects of drug-exposure. The current study is therefore an important contribution in the exploration of long-term developmental deficits of cocaine-exposed and foster children in that it also suggests directions for additional work. Through longitudinal design and multiple site collaboration, future studies need to track large numbers of prenatally exposed and non-exposed infants from birth to their school-aged years to pinpoint long-term differences and similarities.

CONCLUSION

Scant research is available that documents what, if any, deficits are caused by prenatal cocaine exposure in the period beyond infancy. Treatment and prevention strategies for problems associated with drug exposure are dependent on an accurate understanding of the nature and effects of the exposure. Assuming that the deficiencies drug-exposed children manifest are solely a result of the drug-exposure, rather than the surrounding environment, may misguide our intervention efforts. The present study suggests that the pre- and postnatal environment and lifestyle of the drug-abusing parent, much like that of the abusive or neglectful parent, may be associated with factors that adversely influence the children's development perhaps more than the actual drug exposure. Further research is needed to determine the relative impact of each of these factors and thereby to direct our intervention strategies toward reducing the incidence and effects of prenatal drug-exposure on children.

REFERENCES

1. Newborg J, Stack, Wnek L, Guidubaldi J, Svinicki J. *Battelle Developmental Inventory: Examiner's Manual.* Dallas:DLM/Teaching Resources;1984.

2. Hochstadt N, Jaudes P, Zimo D, Schachter J. The medical and psychosocial needs of children entering foster care. *Child Abuse and Neglect.* 1987;11:53-62.

3. McIntyre A, Keesler Y. Psychological disorders among foster children. *Journal of Clinical Child Psychology.* 1986;15:297-303.

4. White R, Benedict M, Jaffe S. Foster child health care supervision policy. *Child Welfare.* 1987;66:387-398.

5. Cooper C, Peterson N, Meier J. Variables associated with disrupted placement in a select sample of abused and neglected children. *Child Abuse and Neglect.* 1987;11:75-86.

6. Goldstein J, Freud A, Solnit A. *Beyond the Best Interests of the Child.* New York, NY: Macmillan Publishing Company; 1973.

7. Fein E. Issues in foster family care: Where do we stand? *American Journal of Orthopsychiatry.* 1991;61:578-583.

8. McIntyre A, Lounsbury K, Berntson D, Steel H. Psychosocial characteristics of foster children. *Journal of Applied Developmental Psychology.* 1988;9:125-137.

9. Benedict M, White R, Stallings R, Cornely D. Racial differences in health care utilization among children in foster care. *Children and Youth Services Review.* 1989;11:285-297.

10. Klee L, Halfon N. Mental health care for foster children in California. *Child Abuse and Neglect.* 1987;11:63-74.

11. Hulsey TC, White R. Family characteristics and measures of behavior in foster and nonfoster children. *American Journal of Orthopsychiatry.* 1989;59:502-509.

12. Singer L, Farkas K, Kliegman R. Childhood medical and behavioral consequences of maternal cocaine use. *Journal of Pediatric Psychology.* 1992;17:389-406.

13. Chasnoff IJ, Landress H, Baret M. The prevalence of illicit drug or alcohol use during pregnancy and discrepancies in mandatory reporting in Pinellas County, Florida. *New England Journal of Medicine.* 1990;322:1202-1206.

14. Gillogley K, Evans A, Hansen R, Samuels S, Batra K. The perinatal impact of cocaine, amphetamine, & opiate use detected by universal intrapartum screening. *American Journal of Obstetrics and Gynecology.* 1990;163:1535-1542.

15. Bingol N, Fuchs M, Diaz V, Stone RK, Gromisch D. Teratogenicity of cocaine in humans. *Journal of Pediatrics.* 1987;110:93-96.

16. Chasnoff IJ, Griffith D, MacGregor S, Dirkes K, Burns K. Temporal patterns of cocaine use in pregnancy. *Journal of the American Medical Association.* 1989;261:1741-1744.

17. Hume R, O'Donnell K, Stanger C, Killam A, Gingras J. In utero cocaine exposure: Observations of fetal behavioral state may predict neonatal outcome. *American Journal of Obstetric Gynecology.* 1989;161:685-690.

18. MacGregor S, Keith L, Chasnoff IJ, Rosner M, Chisum G, Shaw P, Minogue J. Cocaine use during pregnancy: Adverse perinatal outcome. *American Journal of Obstetric Gynecology.* 1987;157:686-690.

19. Young S, Vosper H, Philips S. Cocaine: Its effects on maternal and child health. *Pharmacotherapy.* 1992;12:2-17.

20. Chasnoff I, Griffith D, Freier C, Murray J. Cocaine/polydrug use in pregnancy: Two-year follow-up. *Pediatrics.* 1989;89:284-289.

21. Doberczak T, Shanzer S, Senie R, Kendell S. Neonatal neurologic and electroencephalographic effects of intrauterine cocaine exposure. *The Journal of Pediatrics.* 1988;113:354-358.

22. Brazelton TB. *Neonatal Behavioral Assessment Scale.* 2nd Ed. Philadelphia: JB Lippincott; 1984.

23. Chasnoff IJ, Schnoll K, Burns K, Burns W. Maternal substance abuse during pregnancy: Effects on infant development. *Neurobehavioral Toxicology and Teratology.* 1984;6:277-280.

24. Kaltenbach K, Finnegan L. Prenatal narcotic exposure: Perinatal and developmental effects. *Neurotoxicology.* 1989;10:597-604.

25. Boyd R, Welge P, Sexton P, Miller J. Concurrent validity of the Battelle Developmental Inventory: Relationship with the Bayley Scales in young children with known or suspected disabilities. *Journal of Early Intervention.* 1989;13:14-23.

26. Sexton D, McLean M, Boyd R, Thompson B, McCormick K. Criterion-related validity of a new standardized developmental measure for use with infants who are handicapped. *Measurement and Evaluation in Counseling and Development.* 1988;21:16-24.

27. Finkelhor D. *Child Sexual Abuse: New Theory and Research.* New York, NY: The Free Press; 1984.

28. Helfer R, Kempe R. *The Battered Child: Fourth Edition.* Chicago: University of Chicago Press; 1987.

29. Straus M, Gelles R, Steinmetz S. *Behind Closed Doors: Violence in the American Family.* Newbury Park, CA: Sage Publications; 1980.

Assessment
of Fetal Knee Angular Velocity
as a Possible Method to Determine
the Effect of Prenatal Exposure to Cocaine

Cheryl Riegger-Krugh
Angela Blair
Joyce W. Sparling

SUMMARY. Measurement of fetal joint angular velocity may be beneficial in assessing the effect on the fetus of maternal use of drugs. The effect of maternal cocaine and other drug use on the fetus is not well defined. The ability to measure the effect of maternal drug use on the fetus in a safe, accurate, and reliable way is challenging. A method of measuring fetal knee joint angular velocity is described. Clinical implications for use of the method are discussed. *[Article copies available from The Haworth Document Delivery Service: 1-800-342-9678. E-mail address: getinfo@haworth.com]*

Cheryl Riegger-Krugh, ScD, PT, is Assistant Professor, Program in Physical Therapy, University of Colorado. Angela Blair was in entry-level physical therapy training at the University of North Carolina at Chapel Hill when this study was completed. At present, she is Staff Physical Therapist, Mercy Hospital Charlotte, NC. Joyce W. Sparling, PhD, PT, OT, is Associate Professor Division of Physical Therapy, University of North Carolina at Chapel Hill. She is Project Director for the Maternal and Child Health Postgraduate Training Grant.

Address correspondence to Cheryl Riegger-Krugh, ScD, PT, Program in Physical Therapy, University of Colorado Health Science Center, C244 H200, East 9th Avenue, Denver, CO 80262.

[Haworth co-indexing entry note]: "Assessment of Fetal Knee Angular Velocity as a Possible Method to Determine the Effect of Prenatal Exposure to Cocaine." Riegger-Krugh, Cheryl, Angela Blair, and Joyce W. Sparling. Co-published simultaneously in *Physical & Occupational Therapy in Pediatrics* (The Haworth Press, Inc.) Vol. 16, No. 1/2, 1996, pp. 173-186; and: *Children with Prenatal Drug Exposure* (ed: Lynette S. Chandler, and Shelly J. Lane) The Haworth Press, Inc., 1996, pp. 173-186. Single or multiple copies of this article are available from The Haworth Document Delivery Service [1-800-342-9678, 9:00 a.m. - 5:00 p.m. (EST). E-mail address: getinfo@haworth.com].

© 1996 by The Haworth Press, Inc. All rights reserved.

BACKGROUND

The effect of maternal cocaine use or other drug exposure on the fetus is an important area of public health.[1] The use of drugs by the mother may affect the fetus in a number of ways. Fetal movement is one aspect of the function and behavior of the fetus which could be used safely to determine ill effects of maternal cocaine or other drug use on the fetus. Specifically, if the speed of joint movements is related to a detrimental level of cocaine exposure in fetuses, measurement of fetal joint angular velocity may be particularly useful.

Over the last decade, there has been a dramatic increase in the use of cocaine in general[2,3] and in pregnant women[3,4,5,6,7] in their 20s and 30s.[8] Cocaine use can result in numerous effects on the maternal user[1, 9,10,11,12] and on the newborn. Long-term effects on children of cocaine-using pregnant women has not been documented.

The potential for maternal cocaine use to affect the fetus exists, because cocaine is highly water and lipid soluble and crosses most biologic membranes, including those in the placenta and the fetal blood-brain barrier.[1,7,11,12] An estimated 20% of maternal cocaine is delivered to the fetus.[7] Fetal cocaine is metabolized into norcocaine, an active metabolite with a high level of central nervous system penetration.[3,7] Norcocaine does not readily pass back into the mother's system, but instead becomes incorporated into the amniotic fluid by way of the fetal urine. With ingestion of the amniotic fluid, the fetus is re-exposed to the norcocaine. The exposure to the norcocaine is prolonged even further because the fetal liver is functionally immature and is not able to excrete the drug as quickly as the maternal system.[1,7,9,13] Norcocaine exposure of the fetus may last as long as five or six days after maternal cocaine use.[3,7]

The effects of cocaine on movement performance of the fetus are surmised for the most part from the observation of neonates, who have been exposed before birth. Effects noted in some neonates exposed before birth include tremulousness, irritability, high-pitched crying, and excessive startles.[5] Although additional research has provided some evidence for other problems, including increased incidence of congenital skeletal, ophthalmic, urogenital, cardiac, and nervous system anomalies;[4,7,9,10] asymmetrical growth retardation and lowbirth weight;[9,10] limb reduction deficits;[14] small neonatal head circumference,[15](which may be indicative of impaired fetal brain growth); limited neonatal interaction with caregivers; and diminished state organization,[3,4] the data are inconclusive.

Possible mechanisms by which cocaine results in neonatal effects from fetal exposure include toxicity related to the vasoconstrictive properties of the drug,[9,10,14] impaired transfer of nutrients available to the mother,[18] or some as yet unknown mechanism. Vitamin deficiencies and neglect by mothers of the prenatal state cannot be ruled out as possible indirect effects on the fetus and neonate.[2,4,16] A single exposure to cocaine in the first trimester may be sufficient to place the fetus at risk for neurologic and behavioral deficits.[7] Unfortunately, there appears to be no documented benefit to the neonate of stopping maternal use of cocaine after the first trimester.[17]

Poor state organization and signs of fetal intoxication, such as decreased size of the fetus, have been documented with ultrasound imaging in viable fetuses of mothers using cocaine.[16,18] Integrated video-computer technology and real-time ultrasound now exist at a level of sophistication that allows assessment of fetal movement.[19,20] Ultrasound imaging of the fetus is considered safe without risk to the fetus when used according to American Institute of Ultrasound in Medicine procedures.[21,22]

Fetal movement has been assessed by clinicians and researchers for the purpose of establishing normal age-specific fetal movement and detecting non-characteristic movement at different gestational ages.[20,23-28] Sparling and colleagues developed a fetal movement classification system, the Qualitative Assessment of Fetal Movement (Q-MOVE scale), which includes mostly qualitative and some quantitative measures of fetal movement.[25] The Q-MOVE is used to assess fetal movement in terms of space, time, and force quality measures. Force quality is a qualitative measure of apparent degree of force production, based on relative magnitudes of segmental mass and qualitative assessment of speed of movement.

With maternal use of cocaine, joint movement of the fetus may be slowed or quickened, as both heightened and depressed organizational states relative to movement have been documented in cocaine-exposed fetuses.[5] A quantitative measurement of velocity of movement, such as joint angular velocity, may allow determination of the effect of maternal use of cocaine on the fetus. Joint angular velocity is the speed of joint rotational motion or angular displacement in one direction. In future studies, comparison of joint angular velocity in the fetus and newborn follow-up measures could lead to prediction of the long-term effect of cocaine exposure. None of the existing scales of fetal movement includes quantitative assessment of fetal joint angular velocity.

Measurement of joint movement from the ultrasound recording is easiest in one of the body's larger joints, from which measurement can be made with surface landmarks as well as specific bony landmarks. The knee joint is the easiest joint from which to detect movement on the ultrasound recording, because of the relatively enhanced view by ultrasound of the borders of the thigh and leg and/or the bony landmarks of the thigh and leg, that are clinically used to measure knee joint position.

The purpose of this study was to establish a method to quantitatively measure fetal knee joint angular velocity and to compare this measurement for one fetus exposed to cocaine with the measurement for one low-risk fetus. Specific research questions were:

1. What procedure is necessary to quantitatively measure fetal knee angular velocity?
2. What is the inter-rater reliability of fetal knee angular velocity measurements obtained from ultrasound imaging?
3. Are the ranges of quantitatively assessed fetal knee angular velocities defined for each qualitatively assessed category of fetal knee angular velocity?
4. What is the difference in fetal knee angular velocity in one cocaine exposed versus one low-risk fetus of the same gestational age?

METHODOLOGY

Subjects

Subjects were live fetuses from 14-19 weeks gestational age (GA), whose mothers volunteered to participate in a study to assess fetal movement. At this age range, spontaneous fetal movement is most easily observed, because the fetus is large enough to visualize and is also small enough to be observed in full view in the ultrasound image. One low-risk fetus was studied at 14 and 18 weeks to establish the protocol for measurement of fetal knee angular velocity (Phases I and II). Two subjects, one cocaine-exposed and a second low-risk fetus, were studied at 19 weeks gestational age to allow use of the established protocol to measure knee angular velocity movements (Phase III).

The subjects' mothers were followed by obstetricians in the Division of Maternal and Fetal Medicine at University of North Carolina (UNC) Hospital System. The mother of the first low-risk fetus (Phases I and II) was white, had a college education, and no other children. The mother of the cocaine-exposed fetus identified herself as cocaine-addicted by self-report and was hospitalized for observation immediately after use of an undetermined amount of cocaine. The mother was Black, 31 years old, had children 13 and 4 years old, and was within the age range of the majority of mothers who use cocaine.[8] She was matched according to age range, education, and occupation to the mother of a subject already enrolled in an ongoing study, the Carolina Collaborative Study. The mother of the second low-risk fetus (Phase III) was Caucasian, 25 years old, and had one child aged 3 years. The mothers of both fetuses serving as subjects in Phase III were working at the time of the ultrasound at 19 weeks, had a high school education, were semi-skilled workers and housewives, and were included in Category 3 related to socioeconomic status based on Hollingshead's Two-Factor Index of Social Position.[29] The mothers of the low-risk fetuses reported no previous exposure to cocaine and were identified as otherwise low-risk for infant mortality and morbidity by their obstetricians.

Instrumentation and Materials

Instrumentation included a Cormetrics Aloka 680 ultrasound imager, 1990 upgrade model with a 3.5 MHz single transducer, that could be used to obtain 25-minute fetal ultrasound imagings. Imagings were recorded on 1/2 inch VHS videotapes. The tapes were analyzed using a Panasonic AG 6300 VCR, a Sony high-resolution monitor, an IBM-AT computer, and the Observational Coding System (OCS) software program developed by Research Triangle Collaborative, Inc. A clear, plastic 4.5 cm hand-held goniometer was used to obtain angular displacement measurements.

Testing Procedure

In accordance with the clinic procedures of the Division of Maternal and Fetal Medicine, interviews were conducted with the subjects' mothers to obtain demographic information and assess existence, amount, and pattern of substance abuse related to cocaine, alcohol, nicotine, marijuana, and other drugs. Free ultrasound imagings for all mothers of subjects were offered as an incentive for participation in the study. Each mother signed an informed consent form. Each mother was followed throughout subject selection, interview, and two ultrasound imagings. Following the final imaging, a copy of the videotape was given to each mother.

Each mother received 25 minutes of ultrasound imaging at University Hospitals. Imagings of the fetus for Phase I and II were conducted at 14 and 18 weeks GA. Imagings of the fetuses for Phase III were conducted at 19 weeks GA. Mothers were semi-recumbent and within view of the imaging monitor during the imagings. During the first five minutes of viewing, the ultrasonographer described fetal position, body parts, and fluid levels. Biparietal diameter and long bone measurements were obtained in order to establish fetal GA. For the remaining 20 minutes, the transducer was positioned to obtain both sagittal and frontal views of the fetal lower limbs. Maintenance of either the sagittal or frontal view was limited by fetal movement and position. Observations were explained to mothers throughout the imagings.

Videotape Analysis Procedure

Videotapes were analyzed in the UNC Observational Research Laboratory. The videotaped imagings were coded to maintain confidentiality and copied with a 100 frame/sec time code for accuracy in obtaining exact coding segments. Measurements of knee flexion and extension in degrees were obtained by placing the goniometer directly on the screen of the viewing monitor. To calculate angular displacement, angles of knee flexion/extension were measured, based on specific criteria, for a time interval in seconds to two decimal places. Angular velocity, which is angular displacement/time interval, was then determined in degrees/second. The Q-MOVE scale was used by a skilled independent rater, who was blind to angular velocity measurements, to qualitatively assess knee angular velocity as slow, moderately slow, moderate, moderately fast, or fast. On a range from the slowest to the fastest observed fetal motion, qualitative movements have been categorized as slow, moderately slow, moderate, moderately fast, and fast.[25]

Phase I. A method to determine the anatomical landmarks used for knee flexion/extension position measures was required because bony landmarks, used in standardized measurement of knee position, were not always visible. Comparison of measurements by two testers without determining the landmarks for goniometric measurement was unacceptably poor. During Phase I, each of two testers measured knee joint position before advancing the videotape. The knee joint position in degrees was determined by the following landmarks:

1. the angle formed by the intersection of the midline of the thigh and the midline of the leg, if the external surfaces of the thigh and leg were viewed easily; or
2. the angle formed by the femur, if the external surfaces of the thigh were not viewed easily, and the fibula, if the external surfaces of the leg were not viewed easily.

Using the same goniometer, each investigator independently took three joint angle measurements at the start and at the end of each time interval.

Phase II. During Phase II, the same two testers took independent measurements of the knee angular displacement during an agreed upon time segment. The inclusion criteria for usable videotaped segments were developed during this phase. Segments of videotape were considered acceptable for use in quantifying knee angular velocity if:

1. the view of the fetal lower limb was oriented perpendicular by visual perception to the ultrasound head (and therefore to the investigator);
2. the view of the fetal lower limb (both thigh and leg) was continuous and not disrupted at any time during the movement;
3. the knee movement was continuous during the selected time interval; and
4. the knee movement did not change directions at any point during the selected time interval.

Inter-rater reliability of independent measurements by two testers was assessed during Phase II. Joint angle measurements were made independently by two testers using the criteria for locating knee joint position for an established time interval. Videotapes were initially viewed in real time to allow orientation to the position and general movement of the fetus. Tapes were then viewed frame by frame to determine the start and end angles of knee position for the selected time interval. Each investigator adjusted the videotaped image of the fetal lower limb to eye level to prevent perspective error. The knee position was estimated initially as the investigator viewed the fetal lower limb from a distance of two to three feet. Using the same goniometer, each investigator took three joint angle measurements of the estimated angles at the start and at the end of each time interval. The duration of the movement was determined by subtracting the time at the start from the time at the end of the time interval.

Phase III. Portions of the videotaped movement of one fetus who was cocaine-exposed and one low-risk fetus were determined as acceptable, based on the inclusion criteria. The time interval was agreed upon by the two testers. The assessment of the ultrasound imagings was a blind review. Because the angular position was established by frame by frame analysis of joint position, the duration of the movement was not a limiting factor for quantitative analysis. Each investigator took three independent measurements of knee flexion/extension position at the start and at the end times and calculated angular velocity for the three sets of measurements.

The fetal knee movement for the same subjects was assessed qualitatively and assigned to a category of slow, moderately slow, moderate, moderately fast, or fast velocity from the Q-MOVE scale by viewing the movement in real time.[25] Duration of fetal movement of .5 seconds was required for this qualitative assessment.

Data Reduction

Three knee angular measurements per investigator were averaged to obtain a mean initial or start angle (ϕ_i) and a mean final or end angle(ϕ_f) for each movement. The angular displacement was defined as the absolute difference between the mean initial and mean final angle for each of the three measurements. Mean angular velocity was calculated by dividing the absolute angular displacement by the duration in seconds of each measurement according to the following formula:

$$\varpi = \left| \frac{\sum \frac{\phi_f}{3} - \frac{\phi_i}{3}}{\Delta t} \right|$$

ϖ = mean angular velocity in degrees/second

ϕ_f = angle at the end of the movement in degrees

ϕ_i = angle at the start of the movement in degrees

Δt = duration of the movement in seconds

A combined mean velocity was calculated by averaging the mean angular velocity obtained by each of the two testers. The combined mean velocity was then compared to the qualitative velocity assessment.

Inter-rater reliability of mean angular velocity calculations was determined using the Pearson Correlation Coefficient and the Mann-Whitney U test. Mean and range of angular velocity between the two testers were determined for all measurements in Phase I, II, and III. This was accomplished as each tester independently measured knee angular displacement over the time frame initially agreed upon by the two testers. Calculation of angular velocity was determined by angular displacement/time. The three measures of angular velocity were averaged. The values of the averaged angular velocities were used to determine reliability.

Twenty taped segments were assessed in Phase I. Twenty-eight taped segments were assessed in Phase II. Six and four taped segments were compared in Phase III for the subjects who were cocaine-exposed and low-risk, respectively. These segments represented the totality of usable videotaped fetal knee movement for the subjects in this study.

RESULTS

Fetal knee joint angular velocity can be quantitatively assessed with a high degree of reliability. Inter-rater reliability for Phase I was r = .999 (differences between raters were not significant), for Phase II was r = .989 (not significant), and for Phase III was r = .998 (not significant). All values used to determine the averages and ranges for angular velocity in Table 1 for Phase I, II, and III were used to determine reliability.

Mean differences in averaged knee angular velocities between two testers were calculated (Table 1). Measurements differed from 0.6 degrees/ second in Phases I and III to 19.2 degrees/second in Phase II. On average, velocity measurements by the two testers differed by no more than 5.0 degrees/second in any phase of the study.

Ranges of the averaged fetal knee angular velocities, which were categorized into one of the five qualitative velocity categories of the Q-MOVE scale are listed in Table 2. Calculated knee angular velocities ranged from 11-185 degrees/second. Each of the five qualitatively assessed velocity categories contained a value or range of quantified angular velocity that was distinct from any other category and that increased appropriately with qualitative label.

For the few scorable segments of videotape available for analysis in Phase III, the fetus exposed to cocaine moved at a slower velocity than the low-risk fetus at 19 weeks GA (Table 3). This observation was most dramatic at the fastest qualitatively assessed angular velocity.

DISCUSSION

Research Question 1. What procedure is necessary to quantitatively measure fetal knee angular velocity? A procedure to quantitatively measure fetal knee angular velocity was developed. This method included

TABLE 1. Difference in Fetal Knee Angular Velocity Measures Between Two Testers

PHASE	MEAN DIFFERENCE IN ANGULAR VELOCITY (degrees/second)	RANGE OF DIFFERENCE IN ANGULAR VELOCITY (degrees/second)
I	3.9	0.6 - 6.7
II	5.0	0.7 - 19.2
III	3.2	0.6 - 8.4

TABLE 2. Comparison of Qualitatively Assessed Fetal Knee Angular Velocity to Range of Quantitatively Assessed Fetal Knee Angular Velocity

CATEGORY OF QUALITATIVELY ASSESSED KNEE ANGULAR VELOCITY	VALUE OR RANGE OF QUANTITATIVELY ASSESSED KNEE ANGULAR VELOCITY (in degrees/second)
SLOW	11 - 38
MODERATELY SLOW	NONE ASSESSED
MODERATE	44 - 97
MODERATELY FAST	115
FAST	185

TABLE 3. Comparison of Fetal Knee Angular Velocity in One Cocaine Exposed and One Low-Risk Fetus at 19 Weeks Gestation

VELOCITY MEASURE (degrees/second)	FETUS EXPOSED TO COCAINE	FETUS WITH LOW RISK
MEAN ANGULAR VELOCITY (S.D.)	65.0 + / − 41.1	100.76 + / − 70.6
SLOWEST QUALITATIVELY ASSESSED ANGULAR VELOCITY	28.7	30.7
FASTEST QUALITATIVELY ASSESSED ANGULAR VELOCITY	123.0	229.2

identifying anatomic landmarks for goniometric measurement, using the goniometer to make the measurements, and using inclusion criteria for usable videotaped segments. We estimate that training a person in use of this procedure should require one to two days for a person experienced in viewing fetal movement and five days for an inexperienced viewer. This study represents the first documented attempt known to the authors at development of a procedure for quantifying fetal joint angular velocity.

Research Question 2. What is the inter-rater reliability of fetal knee angular velocity measurements obtained from ultrasound imaging? By following the established procedure for measuring fetal knee angular velocity, two testers were able to take measurements with a reliability of r = .989 with no statistical difference between them. The average difference in velocity of 3.2 (.6-8.4) degrees/second between testers during Phase III movements is a clinical marker of expected velocity differences between two trained testers. Differences of 3.2 degrees or less would be considered insignificant differences if angular velocities were determined by two independent testers.

Research Question 3. Are the ranges of quantitatively assessed fetal knee angular velocities defined for each qualitatively assessed category of fetal knee angular velocity? Each of the five qualitatively assessed velocity categories contained a value or range of quantified angular velocity that was distinct from any other category. In this sense, the quantitative results of angular velocity validate the qualitatively assessed categories as previously established.[25] The number of usable videotape segments was very limited, however, and the angular velocities included in the videotaped segments did not include the whole continuum of angular velocities. Many values within the total range of fetal knee angular velocity remain for which qualitative assessments have not been made. For these preliminary data, the ranges of quantitatively assessed velocities are defined for each qualitatively assessed velocity category.

Research Question 4. What is the difference in fetal knee angular velocity in one fetus who was cocaine-exposed versus one fetus of the same gestational age with low-risk? The one fetus in this study who was exposed to cocaine moved with slower knee angular velocities than the one low-risk fetus. The mean knee angular velocity, angular velocity for slowest qualitatively assessed angular velocity, and angular velocity for the fastest qualitatively assessed angular velocity were all slower for the fetus who was cocaine-exposed. The measures for the slowest qualitatively assessed angular velocity differed by 2 degrees/second, while the measures for the mean angular velocity and the fastest qualitatively assessed angular velocity differed by 35 degrees/second and 106 degrees/second, respectively. The possibility exists that the slowest angular velocities of cocaine-exposed and low-risk subjects are similar, while the fastest angular velocity of those who are cocaine-exposed is much slower than that of low-risk fetuses.

Lester[5] reported both heightened and depressed movement related to organizational states for fetuses who were cocaine-exposed. Maternal use of cocaine may result in increased joint angular velocity for any one fetus under some circumstances and decreased joint angular velocity under other circumstances. Maternal cocaine use may not result in consistently faster or slower joint movement. No conclusion is made by the authors at this time because of the limited number of subjects and limited number of usable videotaped segments.

Limitations of the Study

1. Few videotaped segments met the inclusion criteria. This may be due to time limitation of the ultrasound imaging and eligibility criteria for acceptable videotaped segments.
2. This population and the parents of this population are highly variable. All known and possible confounding variables about the mothers, fetuses, and fathers are difficult to ascertain in this population.

Implications for Further Study

Recommended studies for the future include:

1. establishing norms for the continuum of qualitative and quantitative fetal joint angular velocities in low-risk fetuses of differing gestational age;
2. comparing the norms to qualitative and quantitative fetal joint angular velocities in fetuses exposed to cocaine or other drugs or in fetuses with other pathologies;
3. determining the confounding variables involved for the mother, father, and fetus related to interpreting fetal joint angular velocity; and
4. determining the usefulness of fetal joint angular velocity assessment for prediction of the long-term effect of maternal cocaine or other drug use on the fetus.

CONCLUSIONS

1. Fetal knee angular velocity can be inexpensively assessed with intra-rater reliability of .989 for two trained testers. These quantitative assessments are consistent with findings from qualitative ratings.
2. With preliminary assessment from two subjects, the authors suggest that a cocaine exposure may result in slower knee angular velocities than those of a low-risk fetus. If these results are supported by further research, then extremes of joint angular velocity may be useful in distinguishing risk status of fetuses.

REFERENCES

1. Neuspiel DR, Hamel SC. Cocaine and infant behavior. *J Dev Behav Ped.* 1991;12:55-64.

2. Ryan L, Ehrlich S, Finnegan L. Cocaine abuse in pregnancy: effects on the fetus and newborn. *Neurotoxicol Teratol.* 1987; 9:295-299.

3. Schneider JW, Griffith DR, Chasnoff IJ. Infants exposed to cocaine in utero: implications for developmental assessment and intervention. *Infants and Young Children.* 1989; 2:25-36.

4. Chasnoff IJ, Burns WJ, Schnol SH, Burns KA. Cocaine use in pregnancy. *N Engl J Med.* 1985;313:666-669.

5. Lester BM, Corwin MJ, Sepkoski C et al. Neurobehavioral syndromes in cocaine-exposed newborn infants. *Child Dev.* 1991;62:694-705.

6. Lia-Hoagberg B, Knoll K, Swaney S et al. Relationship of street drug use, hospitalization, and psychosocial factors to low birthweight among low-income women. *Birth.* 1988;15:8-13.

7. Nair BS, Watson RR. Cocaine and the pregnant woman. *J Reprod Med.* 1991;36:862-867.

8. Chapman JK, Worthington LA, Cook MJ, Mayfield PW. Cocaine-exposed infants: a potential generation of at-risk and vulnerable children. *Infant-Todd Interven.* 1992;2(3):223-237.

9. Bandstra ES, Burkett G Maternal-fetal and neonatal effects of in utero cocaine exposure. *Sem Perinat.* 1991;15:288-301.

10. Bingol N, Fuchs M, Diaz V et al. Teratogenicity of cocaine in humans. *J Pediatr.* 1987; 110:93-96.

11. Bresnahan K, Brooks C, Zuckerman BS. Prenatal cocaine use: impact on infants and mothers. *Ped Nursing.* 1991;17:123-129.

12. Farrar HC, Kearns GL. Cocaine: clinical pharmacology and toxicology. *J Pediatr.* 1989;115:665-675.

13. Burkett G, Yasin S, Palow D. Perinatal implications of cocaine exposure. *J Reprod Med.* 1990;35:35-42.

14. Hoyme HE, Jones KL, Dixon SD et al. Prenatal cocaine exposure and fetal vascular disruption. *Pediatr.* 1990;85:743-747.

15. Zuckerman B, Frank DA, Hingson R et al. Effects of maternal marijuana and cocaine use on fetal growth. *N Engl J Med.* 1989;320:762-768.

16. Hume RF, O'Donnell KJ, Stanger CL et al. In utero cocaine exposure: observations of fetal behavioral state may predict neonatal outcome. *Am J Obstet Gynecol.* 1989;161:685-690.

17. Chasnoff IJ, Griffity DR, MacGregor S et al. Temporal patterns of cocaine use in pregnancy: perinatal outcome. *JAMA.* 1989;261:1741-1744.

18. Frank DA, Bauchner H, Parker S et al. Neonatal body proportionality and body composition after in utero exposure to cocaine and marijuana. *J Pediatr.* 1990;117:622-626.

19. Seeds JW, Cefalo RC. *Practical Obstetric Ultrasound.* Rockville, MD: Aspen; 1986.

20. Sparling JW, Wilhelm IJ. Quantitative measurement of fetal movement: Fetal-posture and movement assessment (F-PAM). In: Sparling JW ed. *Concepts in Fetal Movement Research*. Binghamton, NY: The Haworth Press, Inc.; 1993:97-114.

21. Tucker LB, Gentry WR, Thomas EA, Sparling JW. Ultrasound safety: A descriptive study of the potential effects of early imaging. In: Sparling JW ed. *Concepts in Fetal Movement Research*. Binghamton, NY: The Haworth Press, Inc.; 1993:77-95.

22. American Institute of Ultrasound in Medicine. Bioeffects considerations for the safety of diagnostic ultrasound. *J Ultrasound Med.* 1988;7:S1-38.

23. deVries JIP, Visser GHA, Prechtl HFR. The emergence of fetal behaviour. I. Qualitative aspects. *Early Hum Dev.* 1982;7:301-322.

24. deVries JIP, Visser GHA, Prechtl HFR. The emergence of fetal behaviour. II. Quantitative aspects. *Early Hum Dev.* 1985;12:99-120.

25. Green S, Sparling JW. Q-MOVE: qualitative assessment of fetal movement. In: Sparling JW ed. *Concepts in Fetal Movement Research*. Binghamton, NY: The Haworth Press, Inc.; 1993:115-137.

26. Ianniruberto A, Tajani E. Ultrasonographic study of fetal movements. *Semin Perinatol.* 1981;5(2):175-181.

27. Prechtl HFR. Qualitative changes of spontaneous movements in fetus and preterm infant are a marker of neurological dysfunction. *Early Hum Dev.* 1990;23:151-158.

28. Riegger-Krugh CL. Relationship of mechanical and movement factors to prenatal musculoskeletal development. In: Sparling JW ed. *Concepts in Fetal Movement Research*. Binghamton, NY: The Haworth Press, Inc.; 1993:19-37.

29. Hollingshead, AB. *The Two-Factor Index of Social Position*. New Haven: privately published, 1975.

Index

Page numbers followed by f indicate figures; page numbers followed by t indicate tables.

Aboagyne, K., 116
Abortion
conflicting rights issues and, 10
effect on child health and
maternal responsibility, 12
Adamitis, S.M., 68
Adolescent(s)
alcohol use in, prevalence, 111
marijuana use in, prevalence, 111
pregnancy in
alcohol use during, effects on
offspring, 115
complications of prenatal
substance use on, 111-128
Pittsburgh study, 116-123.
See also under
Pittsburgh study
effects on children, 112-113
effects on mother, 113-114
infants with low birth rate due
to, 112
marijuana use during, effects
on offspring, 115-116
obstetric complications due to,
113-114
prevalence, 111
tobacco use during, effects on
offspring, 114-115
smoking among, prevalence, 111
Adversarial rights-based model,
critique of, 8-10
Akbari, H.M., 25
Alcohol. *See also* Substance abuse

prenatal exposure to, jitteriness
due to, 41
Alcohol use
during adolescent pregnancies,
effects on offspring, 115,119
in adolescents, prevalence, 111
during pregnancy, effects on
infants and young children,
54
Alessandri, S.M., 68
Alpert, J., 116
Amaro, H., 114,116
Analyses of covariance (ANCOVAs),
in assessment of motor
behavior in children
following prenatal drug
exposure, 98
Anderson, G.M., 24
Anemia, in adolescent mothers, 113
Angelopoulos, J., 134
Anxiety, in substance abusers, 56
Arendt, R., 134
Aten, M.A., 67
Autonomy, defined, 8
Azmitia, E.C., 25

Balance, in assessment of motor
behavior in children
following prenatal drug
exposure, 96
Bandstra, E., 139
Barzelay, D., 22

© 1996 by The Haworth Press, Inc. All rights reserved. *187*

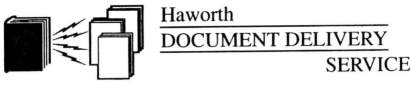

Haworth
DOCUMENT DELIVERY
SERVICE

This valuable service provides a single-article order form for any article from a Haworth journal.

- *Time Saving:* No running around from library to library to find a specific article.
- *Cost Effective:* All costs are kept down to a minimum.
- *Fast Delivery:* Choose from several options, including same-day FAX.
- *No Copyright Hassles:* You will be supplied by the original publisher.
- *Easy Payment:* Choose from several easy payment methods.

Open Accounts Welcome for . . .
- Library Interlibrary Loan Departments
- Library Network/Consortia Wishing to Provide Single-Article Services
- Indexing/Abstracting Services with Single Article Provision Services
- Document Provision Brokers and Freelance Information Service Providers

---

MAIL or *FAX* THIS ENTIRE ORDER FORM TO:

Haworth Document Delivery Service
The Haworth Press, Inc.
10 Alice Street
Binghamton, NY 13904-1580

or FAX: 1-800-895-0582
or CALL: 1-800-342-9678
9am-5pm EST

PLEASE SEND ME PHOTOCOPIES OF THE FOLLOWING SINGLE ARTICLES:

1) Journal Title: _____
   Vol/Issue/Year: _____ Starting & Ending Pages: _____
   Article Title: _____
   _____

2) Journal Title: _____
   Vol/Issue/Year: _____ Starting & Ending Pages: _____
   Article Title: _____
   _____

3) Journal Title: _____
   Vol/Issue/Year: _____ Starting & Ending Pages: _____
   Article Title: _____
   _____

4) Journal Title: _____
   Vol/Issue/Year: _____ Starting & Ending Pages: _____
   Article Title: _____
   _____

(See other side for Costs and Payment Information)

COSTS: Please figure your cost to order quality copies of an article.

1. Set-up charge per article: $8.00
   ($8.00 × number of separate articles) _____
2. Photocopying charge for each article:
   1-10 pages: $1.00 _____

   11-19 pages: $3.00 _____

   20-29 pages: $5.00 _____

   30+ pages: $2.00/10 pages _____

3. Flexicover (optional): $2.00/article _____
4. Postage & Handling: US: $1.00 for the first article/
   $.50 each additional article _____

   Federal Express: $25.00 _____

   Outside US: $2.00 for first article/
   $.50 each additional article _____

5. Same-day FAX service: $.35 per page _____

GRAND TOTAL: _____

METHOD OF PAYMENT: (please check one)
❏ Check enclosed   ❏ Please ship and bill. PO # _____
(sorry we can ship and bill to bookstores only! All others must pre-pay)
❏ Charge to my credit card: ❏ Visa; ❏ MasterCard; ❏ Discover;
                              ❏ American Express;

Account Number: _____ Expiration date: _____

Signature: ✗ _____

Name: _____ Institution: _____

Address: _____

_____

City: _____ State: _____ Zip: _____

Phone Number: _____ FAX Number: _____

MAIL or *FAX* THIS ENTIRE ORDER FORM TO:

Haworth Document Delivery Service | **or FAX:** 1-800-895-0582
The Haworth Press, Inc. | **or CALL:** 1-800-342-9678
10 Alice Street | 9am-5pm EST)
Binghamton, NY 13904-1580 |